Praise for *The Body Mechanic's Handbook*

You need expert help: "When part of your body breaks down, it may seem to come out of the blue, almost spontaneously. If you decide to dig in and work on understanding what caused the breakdown, you're going to need some expert help. I've seen many of my patients benefit from the system Geoff outlines in the Body Mechanic's Handbook. As you put the pieces of your health puzzle together, you're going to need a great team; I'm glad to have Geoff Dakin on mine. This book can put him on yours."
  – DR. JEFFREY SCHOLTEN BSc DC DCCJP. President of the International Chiropractors Association's Council on Upper Cervical Care. Clinic Director, The Vital Posture™ Clinic. Calgary AB Canada

I did the exercises daily: "After six months of lower back pain, I sent Geoff Dakin an email. I needed help but didn't know what to try. After hearing the description of my symptoms, Geoff sent me a customized version of his exercises. It was amazing that he knew what exercises to suggest, without seeing me in person. Although it wasn't easy the first few days, I did the exercises daily. I was totally amazed that after a couple weeks my pain had improved immensely. I can now bend freely, do chores and sleep without any pain. I can't thank Geoff enough for all the great help. May God bless him always."
  – PAULINE KARIMI. Nairobi Kenya

Alignment First has become a lifestyle: "For eleven years I endured muscle and nerve pain, a vast array of therapies and medications, and was told by many that this was now my life. That's how I spent my 40s. Now, three years after meeting Geoff Dakin, I am completely pain-free, and strength has returned to my left leg. The Alignment First Protocol is more than just a treatment, it has become a lifestyle for my husband and I. At age 59, not only is he touching his toes for the first time since he was a teenager, but his doctor says he's taller than before!"
  – SUSAN SEUFERT. Calgary AB Canada

His Alignment First exercises changed my life: "After suffering an injury over 20 years ago, I was told by numerous medical experts that my chronic pain condition would dictate a future involving therapy and related medical care, probably including surgery. After a multitude of physiotherapists, acupuncturists, massage therapists, chiropractors and doctors couldn't help me, I stumbled across Geoff Dakin. His Alignment First exercises changed my life. After the very first session I was able to sleep through the night for the first time in years. I knew there was hope. The exercises are simple, progressive and target my body's needs. Two years after completing the protocol I am still pain-free and no longer living in fear of it returning."

– PAULINE WAGENAAR. Calgary AB Canada

Alignment First ... is an incredible system: "I was in a bad car vs bicycle accident and immobile for 3 months. Half of my body was working overtime to compensate for my other-sided weakness. Even though I broke my left hip, for a while my right knee hurt worse from overuse and improper use. While on vacation in Canada, I saw Geoff once in his office. I felt great following the stretches and manipulations. He has magic hands, but it truly was his Alignment First Protocol that I took with me that brought me lasting relief. It is an incredible system that I would recommend to anyone."

– DR. BRIAN NEWELL MD. Cleveland Ohio USA

Grateful for the quality of life restored to me: "I was bedridden for almost two years following a serious car accident. I struggled with constant pain and spent several years walking with a cane. I was referred to see Geoff in Mexico, but as I had already seen over 45 medical professionals, I was more than a little skeptical. I ended up extending my stay in Mexico because of the relief I was getting with Geoff's system. I returned to work with him in Cabo two more times over the next year and a half. I will always be grateful for the quality of life Geoff restored to me with his work, caring and dedication."

– AARON MORI. Vernon BC Canada

I haven't felt this good in years: "After a seemingly unending series of small injuries, I was getting concerned that I wasn't going to be able to enjoy my middle and later years without pain. By focusing on the postural and alignment issues that were causing my injuries, Geoff was able to, quite literally, get me straightened out. I haven't felt this good in years."
— MARK THOMPSON. Victoria BC Canada

All reported vast improvement: "I was one of the first scope surgeries on the hip at the Hospital for Special Surgery in New York and had worked with countless physical therapists. Geoff discovered postural issues no other professional had noticed and recommended corrective exercises that had me back to my fitness regimen quickly and without discomfort. I have not had any pain in the years since I worked with Geoff. I've sent many clients suffering from chronic pain to Geoff and all reported vast improvement."
— NICOLE MONTGOMERY. San Jose del Cabo BCS Mexico

Straight forward. Effective. Empowering: "I have endured chronic, debilitating back pain for more than three decades. In recent years, even the normal range of motion required for everyday activities was often out of the question. My activities and mobility became increasingly limited and my best hope was to 'push through' and manage the aftermath with meds and bedrest. That is, until Dr. Gordon Hasick referred me to Geoff Dakin. Geoff's assessment revealed body-wide imbalances and misalignments. So, we began undoing 30 years of dysfunction. Geoff's methods are straight forward, shockingly effective in their simplicity and incredibly empowering in their end result. The simple exercises found in The Body Mechanic's Handbook, done faithfully, have quite literally altered the course of my life. Back pain is a distant memory. I no longer hesitate to participate in activities, old and new. Where I could not bend to pick up small objects before, I am now able to deadlift more than my bodyweight. It is an amazing gift to be able to embrace life and challenge myself physically without fear. Today, thanks to Geoff, the sky's the limit!"
— CATHERINE MUIRHEAD. Calgary AB Canada

Thankful I am: "I have worked for years as a long-distance truck driver, spending many hours a day sitting behind the wheel of a big rig. My health has suffered due to the lack of exercise and continual stress on my body. I cannot express how thankful I am to Geoff Dakin! Because of his Alignment First Protocol, I haven't felt this close to pain-free and enjoyed such flexibility in movement in years. I couldn't be happier. Thank you, Geoff!"

– BRUCE SINCLAIR. Calgary AB Canada

The roadmap for lower back pain sufferers: "I regularly collaborate with Geoff on complex cases and I have seen everything from chronic hip and lower back pain to knee and foot pain problems resolve in patients who have used this protocol. The Body Mechanic's Handbook is a veritable roadmap for lower back pain sufferers looking to regain health and wellbeing."

– DR. JORDAN AUSMUS DC. Calgary AB Canada

Daily stretches keep the problem at bay: "I had been experiencing chronic hip pain for years and had seen countless well-regarded medical experts and therapists. No one was able to provide solutions that lasted, and my pain always returned to the same level very quickly. During the first session with Geoff Dakin, he identified the misalignment problem, helped me shift my pelvis back into alignment and gave me a few daily stretches that seem to keep the problem at bay. I am incredibly grateful as I was starting to feel I was going to have deep hip pain for the rest of my life. One other happy outcome, after he helped me shift my hip alignment back into place, the golf swing I thought was long lost came back and feels great!"

– KATHY STANKIEVECH. Calgary AB Canada

Improvement in pain: "Geoff Dakin's unique brand of exercise therapy is excellent. So many of my patients returned from his office with improvement in their pain, when others had been unable to achieve the same results."

– DR. MIKE ORTH MD. Edmonton AB Canada

Alignment First worked for me: "I injured myself during dance training and the pain was overwhelming. I saw a lot of different doctors and therapists but after seven months, I was still getting around in a wheelchair because of the pain. Nobody I saw knew how to help me or where to begin. After the first session with Geoff, I never took the wheelchair to his office again. In just 3 months I was pain-free. The Alignment First exercises worked for me."

– RACHEL KRISA. Calgary AB Canada

THE BODY

MECHANIC'S
HANDBOOK

Why You Have Low Back Pain and
How to Eliminate It at Home

Second Edition

GEOFF DAKIN

Vitruvian Publishing
Calgary

The Body Mechanic's Handbook
Copyright © 2018 by Geoff Dakin.

First published in 2016 by Vitruvian Publishing.
Second Edition published in 2018 by Vitruvian Publishing.
Second Edition edited by George Roberts.

ISBN: 978-0-9951826-3-9

Printed in the United States of America.

I dedicate this book to the thousands of patients who have entrusted me with their physical wellbeing by allowing me to practice and improve my craft. I also dedicate it to thousands more who will use this book to improve their lives. Though we may never meet in person, we will share back stories of renewed comfort, pain relief and a much better quality of life.

Contents

Foreword

The practice of medicine was transformed in 1828. That's when America's first dental school opened in Ohio. That school turned dentistry into a separate branch of healthcare and helped launch the process of Medical Specialization that continues to this day. As McGill University professor and author, George Weisz, explains, specialization works because it enables "the greater perfection that could be achieved by concentrating on a single field".

But in the process of dividing the body up into its specialized fields, we sometimes lose sight of the fact that the body is a complete and interactive working machine. All the parts are interconnected. And they don't just work together. They rely on each other.

I see this interconnection, every day, as a dentist who treats chronic pain patients. My job is to attend to their teeth and how they function, but my diagnosis and care extends well beyond their jaws. I am keenly aware of how a patient's bite can affect their posture. And I am also very cognizant of how their posture can affect their bite.

So, I was delighted to discover that Geoff Dakin practiced the same kind of "full body press" approach to healthcare that I and Dr. Jeff Scholten, a NUCCA chiropractor, provide to our patients. The three of us now collaborate on behalf of our shared cases because we are committed to optimizing patient care and more importantly, patient outcomes.

Our practice philosophy is well represented, simply explained and sensibly demonstrated, if not proven, in Geoff Dakin's book, *The Body Mechanic's Handbook*. In layperson's terms, he helps his readers understand how all parts of the body influence structural balance. How structural stress and strain leads to muscle fatigue, muscle spasm, ligament and tendon pain and a myriad of other pain patterns. Geoff then offers the reader an alternative to traditional symptom focus with its localized, temporary relief and its pharmacologic interventions.

Why just treat the symptoms of a problem when structural insight can shine a light on the root cause of your problem? Why not learn how to use simple exercises and stretches to lead you away from that problem, out of pain, and hand you back the freedom to enjoy your life?

This is what *The Body Mechanic's Handbook* gives you. The power to change your life.

Dr. Curtis Westersund,
Calgary, Alberta
Dentalife.com

Introduction

"I wrote this book to show you how to use the Alignment
First Protocol to make your lower back pain go away.
And stay away."
— GEOFF DAKIN

The majority of North Americans struggle with back pain. Some estimates suggest 80 percent of us have experienced discomfort. And yet, in spite of billions of dollars spent on researching and treating these problems, the number of sufferers seems to be increasing. So, one has to ask, how is that possible?

Well, if you're like millions of other back pain sufferers, you've probably tried massage, physical therapy and/or chiropractic care. I expect you experienced some temporary relief. But because you're reading this book with back pain in the title, I am assuming you didn't enjoy lasting success.

I expect your lower back continues to hurt. That the pain probably comes and goes. And when it's there, when it takes the joy out of your day, you don't want to move. Or walk. Or sit. Or, if sitting, stand.

It's perverse, is what back pain is. And it's pervasive. It comes without warning. And though it may leave on its own, it's too often not soon enough. Worse, it doesn't stay away. So, you are forced to seek relief, however you can find it.

And I know. That search can be discouraging. You'll hear different stories from various healthcare experts. They're experienced and capable practitioners. They're well intentioned. But they all have their own approach to back pain. And they each tell a different story. So, who do you believe? And how do you not get frustrated and disillusioned? Because that's what I'd be, were I in your shoes.

If what you've read so far strikes a chord, if it sounds similar to what you are experiencing, I wouldn't be surprised to hear that your current, therapeutic strategy includes anti-inflammatory and/or pain medications. Unfortunately, medicating lower back pain doesn't work. It's like putting a band aid over the engine warning light, in your car. It needs service. It's not going to fix itself. So, you have to do the right thing. You have to take it to a mechanic.

Pain is much like that engine warning light. It's your body's way of warning you that something is wrong. Something needs service. To ignore this warning, to try and mask it with drugs, is simply a bad idea. You'll be putting a band aid on something that needs more from you.

Your best bet is to treat lower back pain for what it is: an important signal that has to be properly dealt with. Which is what this book is all about. It provides a protocol you can use to properly alleviate, if not eradicate, that painful signal.

How do I know it works? Since 1989, I've worked with thousands of patients. And most of them told me a variation of this story: "I've had lower back pain for a number of years. X-rays have revealed no obvious structural problem. I have seen various therapists and doctors, but nobody seems to know why I have this pain."

Inevitably, when I assessed these patients' postures, I found that their pelvises were unbalanced or out of alignment. One side of the pelvis was either significantly higher, or tilted further forward, than the other side of the pelvis. To me, it's obvious: if the pelvis is significantly misaligned, the lower back is going to become irritated and complain.

After all, the pelvis is the crux of the body. It functions as the foundation for our upper body. And because our hip joints are located on the pelvis, it is also, in an upside-down way, the foundation for our lower body.

So, it has to be asked: how can any treatment, applied directly to your lower back, make your problem go away and stay away? How can that happen, when the root cause of your problem is the crookedness of your pelvis? I grant you that some misplaced treatments may calm your symptoms temporarily. But that's the most you can hope for, because the world's best techniques applied to the wrong place have no chance of long term success. They're just not going to be effective.

Here's why. The scientific study of pain identifies three components of any pain problem. There is a biological, a psychological and an emotional piece. In this book, I'll discuss the psychological and emotional pieces, but my focus is on eliminating the biological causes of lower back pain.

It's my focus because most of our discomfort is caused when our major weight-bearing joints – ankles, knees and hips – are misaligned. Misalignment creates instability, something our bodies hate. So it tries to compensate. It triggers muscle spasms and it induces bracing postures. It's trying to increase stability. But the muscles, engaged in this process, can only handle the extra work for a while and then they tire out. When that happens, the body has to create additional muscular compensations. These compensations – or counterbalances, if you like – eventually become painful.

The pain can be mild, moderate or severe. It may take hours, days or years before your body is affected enough for you to become aware of it. And though this process is quite common, everyone's experience of it is different.

In an ideal world, your back would be so much happier if you had a perfectly neutral posture. But that would require an environment where your body was only asked to respond to a perfect balance of physical demands, a hundred percent of the time. That's not what happens.

What happens is this. The shape, position and organization of our spine, ribcage and pelvis evolves in response to our on-going muscle activities. So even if, as infants, we developed a perfectly aligned body structure, our active lifestyles provide ample opportunities to accidentally knock it out of kilter. Add to this, the sedentary behaviours that we adopt as we mature, and imbalances are inevitable over time.

Asymmetrical alignment is the result. In fact, misalignment of the skeleton has become so commonplace, it tends to be accepted as the norm. That acceptance is the key problem with most approaches to lower back pain. By accepting misalignment as the norm. By ignoring it and, in effect, hiding the key piece of the pain puzzle in plain sight, many of my well-intentioned colleagues are missing the obvious, root cause of pain.

Here's what happens when alignment is overlooked. Back in 2013, at one of our weekly clinic meetings, I heard about an injured dancer. A teenaged girl who had collapsed, during a dance practice, with acute pain in her right hip. The pain was so severe, she was unable to walk or even to stand comfortably. Indeed, she spent most of her waking hours in a wheelchair. And despite working with a team of medical specialists at a local hospital, her symptoms were getting worse; not better.

As I listened to the particulars of this case, I was reminded of something one of my early mentors, Paul St, John, said years ago. He had described the only type of postural misalignment, that he was aware of, that could cause someone to need a wheelchair. In that case, one side of the pelvis was tilted excessively forward, while the other side of the pelvis was tilted excessively backward.

In over twenty years of practice, I never encountered this condition. I had seen thousands of cases of excessive forward or backward pelvic tilts, where both sides of the pelvis moved in unison or, where one side moved and the other didn't. But to have the two sides of the pelvis tilting excessively in opposite directions! That's rare.

I shared the story of this case with my associates and a couple weeks later, I met Rachel, the dancer. It had been seven months since her injury. She was still in a wheelchair. She was still experiencing the same pain in her right hip, from the very first day of her injury. Additionally, she was now struggling with pains in her back, neck and shoulders.

Imagine my surprise when, during my initial assessment, I discovered that she did indeed have an extreme version of the pelvic misalignment described by my mentor, so many years before!

During that very first session, we had considerable success normalizing her pelvic position. Not only that, but two weeks later, when she arrived at her second session, she did so without her wheelchair. She was using crutches and already experiencing dramatic improvement. Rachel left the fourth session carrying her crutches. Three months later, after eight sessions, she was pain-free.

I share this case with you to highlight the moral of the story. That being: quite a few renowned healthcare experts had worked with Rachel. But they had experienced zero success because assessment of her pelvic position was not part of their procedure. In their worldview, crooked pelvises were either not possible, or not important. So their plan just ignored the alignment piece of the pain puzzle.

I still find their disregard disturbing because, it is generally agreed, the body functions better and more comfortably, when all its major weight-bearing joints are properly aligned. Circulation is better. Muscle tone is improved. And it is literally easier to hold yourself upright against the pull of gravity.

When our joints are misaligned, it's typically due to imbalances in the length and tone of our muscles and other soft tissues. These awkward positions challenge our ability to properly activate muscles in the area in question. This ability, or inability, to control our muscles in a coordinated way, is called motor control. When it's out of whack, we generate dysfunctional patterns of movement. If they become habitual and self-perpetuating, they will lead to chronic pain problems, which can sometimes persist for decades.

And here's the thing: almost all common causes of lower back pain are related to this "out of whack" picture I've just painted for you. They all involve muscle imbalances, misaligned joints and dysfunctional motor control. I know it sounds complicated and, quite frankly, it sometimes is. But there's good news, too: the majority of these problems are identifiable, preventable and correctable.

It is one thing to understand your pain situation. That's your first step towards resolving your discomfort. The other thing you have to understand is, in order to mitigate and/or eradicate your pain, you have to take the appropriate action. You have to be prepared to invest the time and effort required to train your body to become healthy and happy, again.

To achieve this, you need a maintenance program. A daily ritual to remind your body how to become organized, as best it can be. That's why I developed the Alignment First Protocol. It's a system of corrective exercises for self-treatment, that you can perform at home. The protocol leads you through a series of steps designed to re-educate your body. To ease it out of the misaligned postures that are the cause of your chronic back pain. And to make it ever-easier for your body to become straighter, more mobile and more comfortable. Daily practice of the protocol exercises makes all of this this possible.

Know that you don't have to achieve a perfectly neutral posture. It is neither a cure-all, nor is it a requirement, for a pain-free back. However, to strive towards that ideal posture, in a systematic way, is to go down the path that's been proven to improve function and comfort in the body.

Obviously, the protocol is a process. And although some people experience dramatic rapid changes, others are forced to develop their capacities for patience, along the way. We're all so different, it's not surprising that the experience is unique for each of us.

What is common for all of us, however, is the body-learning process of the protocol. It's designed to have you spend more time practicing the exercises that are appropriate for your particular situation, and less time practicing the exercises your body can already perform easily. It's a self-customizing program that helps you develop the daily routine that's best for you and your back.

That's why I called this book The Body Mechanic's Handbook. Many people assume I chose this title because I'm talking about the mechanics of the body. But the fact is, the title actually refers to a person: you. I want you to become your own body mechanic. After all, you know as well as I do, that we should both be performing regular maintenance on our bodies. So that's what the protocol is designed to do. Think of it as an operator's manual. It provides you with the kind of information you need to understand your lower back pain. And then it bolsters your understanding with practical steps that you can take, to become your own body mechanic.

I'm advocating this approach in lieu of following in the tracks of those who are content to manage their joint health through medication and surgery. The body mechanic route is, by far, the better choice. It's non-invasive. It's non-chemical. It's just the body working in harmony with itself. And though no one can promise that you will never need future surgical help, I do know you will accomplish more with the Alignment First Protocol than you might imagine.

Don't wait until your "wheels are falling off". The time to start caring for your muscles and joints is now. Indeed, if you manage your body's mechanical health properly, you may just help your joints last a lifetime. So, keep reading and let me show you how easy it is to become your own, very capable body mechanic.

It's time for the obligatory medical disclaimer. Primum non nocere is a Latin phrase that translates as first, do no harm. Please do check with your doctor before beginning any exercise-based program. The Alignment First Protocol does not place a huge demand on your cardiovascular system but, if your health is compromised to the extent that you are under close medical supervision, please talk to him/her about this program before you start.

I also stress that if you are suffering from chronic debilitating back pain, it is perfectly in order for you to seek out a healthcare practitioner who specializes in the elimination of alignment-related pain problems. The detail and accuracy of assessment and treatment from such a practitioner cannot be reproduced via a do-it-yourself handbook.

If you are exploring the online world of self-care and corrective exercise, I urge you to tread cautiously. Frankly, when I review the lower-back-pain-related videos on YouTube, what I see is often worrisome. There is no shortage of information out there, but for every solid source of information like Dr. Evan Osar DC or Dr. Kelly Starrett PT, there are many questionable sources. Some of these 'how-to videos and blogs' are putting people in harm's way.

For example, if you're suffering from a hyperextended lower back, you are unlikely to find relief with a program that emphasizes loading your lower back in extension. It's like adding fuel to a fire. Conversely, if you're struggling with a lack of lower back extension, a program promoting ab crunches to strengthen your core is more likely to make your problem worse, not better. But enough about what doesn't work.

Let's talk about what does work: The Alignment First Protocol.
If you have already sought professional help for your pain and not experienced any success, this book may be for you. While the protocol is unlikely to result in an overnight, miracle cure of your back, it might. And even if it doesn't, the improvements you make in postural alignment, mobility, strength and comfort will accumulate and stabilize with practice. Indeed, the vast majority of people who commit to this process find it incredibly satisfying, empowering and pain-relieving.

If that sounds like something you'd like to experience, then let's get started.

Name Dropping. In this book, I acknowledge the pioneers, gurus and mentors who inspired me to develop a protocol to relieve chronic lower back pain. Read about these thoughtful practitioners and their therapies and you'll see how they've fostered the concept of structural alignment to enhance our quality of life.

Story Telling. I share a number of client stories as anecdotal illustrations. My intention is to help you see what I'd like you to understand about how you can relieve the pain in your lower back. These stories are not as detailed as case studies, but I expect they will create some rapport between you and my clients' experiences.

REMEMBER:
The good news is that the majority of these problems are identifiable, preventable and correctable.

CHAPTER 1

You Can Do This

"The greatest force in the human body is the natural drive of the body to heal itself – but that force is not independent of the belief system. Everything begins with belief. What we believe is the most powerful option of all."
— NORMAN COUSINS

I chose this quotation because belief – in both yourself and in the therapeutic benefits of gentle exercise – is key to the diminishment and elimination of your lower back pain. And yes, I know, I tread on the fringes of credibility whenever I assure chronic sufferers that a pain-free future is a real possibility for them. But this is not, as my son might say, "crazy talk". Even if you've been suffering for years, it is quite likely you can regain control of your back-pain problem.

In the coming chapters, I'll be asking you to look at yourself – and at your pain and at your body – in a way different from what you've become accustomed to. To begin that transition, you need to open your mind to the prospect of eliminating your lower back pain, in the comfort of your own home. You need to accept that you can experience relief, just like my patient, Pauline, did.

Pauline and I have never met in person, but I had sponsored her, as a little girl, in Kenya. Years later, she found me on Facebook and so we stayed in touch. Then in 2015, she sent a message asking for advice about a back pain she was suffering from. I asked her to describe her symptoms and how they came about. After reviewing them, I sent her a routine of Alignment First exercises. As I expected, she was pain-free within a couple of weeks.

Pauline's story is an excellent example of how the Alignment First Protocol can work as a stand-alone therapy to resolve back pain, without an in-person assessment. Her experience flies in the face of conventional wisdom that continues to try to treat the location of pain – the lower back – even though such misdirected therapies usually don't work.

As mentioned in the Introduction, many of the billions of dollars being spent on back problems, are misdirected at inappropriate care. Too many therapies fail because they endeavour to remedy the symptoms. They don't address the problem. And more often than not, the problem is misalignment.

It just stands to reason: an incorrectly arranged body structure needs to be corrected. To ignore this fact is to waste time and effort on treatments that have close to zero chance of success. No amount of therapy, applied to your lower back, can eliminate your pain in the presence of large, bony alignment problems in your hips and/or pelvis. It's just common sense: if your ankles, knees and hips are out of whack, they have to be brought back into order.

And that applies to all of us, young or old. Earlier, I told you Pauline's story. She's younger than most of the patients I treat in my clinic. Many of them have had their pain problems for a couple years. Others have been searching and suffering for decades. And yet, just like Pauline, once they understand the common causes of lower back pain, it becomes easier to choose how to tackle it. When they realize that asymmetry is their problem, they know that it has to be dealt with.

People chuckle when I say that asymmetry is a bit like alcohol. I say that because your body can tolerate some of it just fine. But too much of it is destabilizing and debilitating. And though alignment perfection is probably an unrealistic goal for most of us, there is magic in the seeking of it. It doesn't really matter whether your bony structure lets you attain alignment perfection or not. The tiny deviations from the theoretical ideal are not the sources of strain that cause chronic back pain. It's the larger deviations that make us hurt.

How do you determine which is which? You don't need a computerized measuring device to detect the asymmetries I am talking about. They're easy enough to see when you know what to look for. Some are even large enough to be recognized by uninterested bystanders. Do you have one shoulder obviously higher than the other? Is one leg shorter than the other? Do your feet point at ten and two instead of straight ahead? These are common alignment problems. If your body is coping successfully with them, it means you're biomechanically inefficient and pain-free — but only for the time being. Eventually, your body will become unable to compensate and cope, at which time you will begin experiencing pain.

Which is why the Alignment First Protocol is designed to help you create the kind of skeletal alignment, balanced muscle tone and mobility that is common in people who have pain-free backs.

To get you there, to help you establish the kind of symmetry you need to become pain-free, I'll be introducing you to a series of exercise progressions. You will be asked to perform them in the sequence described by the protocol. This systematic approach is, essentially, your path to a pain-free back. Indeed, it is the order in which the exercises are done, along with the sum total of their effects, that is the special sauce in this equation.

"I can hardly move! And you want me to exercise?" Yes, I do. But I hasten to point out that many of the exercises require no movement at all. Initially, almost all of the exercises merely require you to relax into a very specific posture. The object is to train your body to be straighter at rest. And then, as bony alignment and muscle balance improve, your body is encouraged to advance through a series of exercise progressions. They will gradually ask more and more of your body but, remember, you are in complete control of the pacing. You'll move from one level to another only when you choose to do so. So don't even try to move with the kind of mobility, skill and strength associated with those who are pain-free. Start slow. Ease into your exercises. And listen to your body. It will guide you towards organizing your physical structure into a comfortable and fairly neutral position, when at rest.

As you will see, most of the exercises that make up the Alignment First Protocol are pretty familiar. What will be new to you, is how the exercise progressions help you gradually improve your structural wellbeing.

There's a variety of these exercise progressions, each aimed at effecting one particular change in your body. This process helps you identify and re-educate your own particular issues. Depending upon your body's needs, the progressions let you adjust the effort required to perform the exercises. This helps you introduce demand at the appropriate level for your current condition. And then, as your body improves, the next exercise in the progression provides an incremental demand that pushes you on, reinforcing that improvement. Over time, these steps prepare your body to make even more changes.

As you follow the instructions for a particular exercise and when you can manage it without experiencing new or increased pain, you can count it as a small victory over your problem. Cherish that victory because your path to a pain-free lower back is going to be built on a collection of such small victories. By way of their accumulation, you'll be helping your body recalibrate itself.

You should know that your body's natural drive to heal itself will not tolerate improper positional changes for long. If it's not comfortable with a change, if your body deems an exercise to be dangerous, it will trigger defense mechanisms. These will either prevent you from performing the exercise or, they will impede the change you are looking for. So, for your efforts to succeed, it's critical that your exercises not be too demanding. On occasion, you may have to find a less onerous exercise in a particular progression or even, temporarily skip one of the exercises in the protocol.

So be patient. Let your body tell you when it's ready to try again. Just listen to your instincts and you'll almost always find ways to modify the exercises enough to enable you to perform and benefit from them.

"Okay, but what if I have a condition?" What if you've been diagnosed with osteoarthritis or degenerative disc disease? Or how about ankylosing spondylitis or spinal stenosis? What then? Well, no matter your diagnosis, you will almost always be better off with a straighter skeleton than a crooked one. To be true, your condition may end up being a limiting factor in terms of how good you can get. But then again, it might not. And since there is no better way to find out than to try, I suggest you do so. Because, more often than not, once the big alignment problems are solved, diagnosed conditions usually turn out to be non-pain-producing.

A couple of cautions. One is, it's not uncommon to encounter stumbling blocks, along the path to a pain-free lower back. You may very well encounter psychological and emotional obstacles related to your personal pain puzzle. And they can be huge for some. So I remind readers that while it is not necessary for them to believe the Alignment First Protocol will eliminate their back pain, it is important that they accept that a decrease in the amount of their pain is, at least, likely. That simple belief, in the possibility of being pain-free, gives you the opportunity to have a successful result.

The other caution is that your motivation can also be a complication. If your pain and the disabilities related to it are somehow rewarding or enriching your life, there are mechanisms within you that may be reluctant to give that up. To overcome this reluctance, you need to want to eliminate your pain for good. That means developing a daily habit of floor exercise in the pursuit of that goal. If that's where you're at, if you can commit to a daily regimen, then keep on reading.

To summarize this chapter: I've emphasized that many people fail to experience success in their search for pain relief because their therapies ignore the importance of bony alignment for a healthy, pain-free lower back. I touched on the Alignment First Protocol and explained how its exercise progressions allow you to customize the exercise demands to match your needs. I also described how the accumulation of tiny exercise victories, over time, will enable you to work your way towards a healthier, happier lower back.

In Chapter 2, I am going to talk about pain and the nervous system, in terms of how they relate to you and the First Alignment Protocol.

REMEMBER:
It's just common sense: if your ankles, knees and hips are out of whack, they have to be brought back into order.

Understanding Pain

"Pain is ready, pain is waiting.
Primed to do its educating"
— DEPECHE MODE

In the movie "As Good as It Gets", the character played by Jack Nicholson got so exasperated he snarled: "I'm drowning here, and you're describing the water!" That scene has become famous because it so perfectly shares the frustration we all experience when someone tells us what we already know. Nicholson was desperate for some helpful insights; but all he got from his friend were platitudes.

That same frustration is felt by chronic pain sufferers when their therapists proclaim: "you have really tight muscles" or "your SI joint is stuck" or "your gluteus medius muscles are weak or won't fire". Like in the movie, these comments are merely "describing the water". All they do is describe symptoms. You already know you're hurting. That's painfully obvious. What you want to know is what's the cause of your chronic pain? And what might be done about it?

And so, to help unravel the mysteries of your chronic issues, we're going to talk about pain itself. It's been my experience that a basic understanding of the subject helps people improve their odds of eliminating their unique problem.

Pain is an enigma, partly because there's so much disagreement amongst the experts. The only thing that most of them agree upon is that there are three major components in any pain problem: biological, psychological and emotional. Historically, the biological causes of pain have received the most attention and thus, the majority of pain-relief efforts. As a result, the healthcare community has developed body-part and technique-specific services for people in pain.

It's no surprise that such specialization produces excellent results with appropriate cases and horrible results with inappropriate ones. But here's the thing: at present, there is no agreed-upon model for matching practitioner specialists with appropriate cases. This missing link is why so many people in pain continue to wander, from one office to another, in search of relief.

The issue is further complicated by some prominent pain-science authors who deny that biomechanical issues are important sources of pain. These authors renounce the structural element and emphasize the psychological and emotional elements of the pain equation to the detriment of all of us in the healthcare community. I find these anti-biomechanical sentiments disturbing because chronic pain is truly a multi-faceted problem. And as you will see throughout this book, biomechanical issues contribute significantly to lower back pain. In fact, I go to great lengths to explain how you can use this knowledge to minimize your own pain problems.

I do acknowledge that an increased emphasis on the psychological and emotional pieces of the pain puzzle has been beneficial. It has led to our pain problems being viewed from a systems perspective, rather than from a location perspective. This systems approach will, I believe, eventually lead to answers for all kinds of pain problems.

And I want to be clear that, while not claiming skeletal alignment to be the end-all and be-all for pain relief, it is a critical component for the treatment of pain in the lower back and everywhere else. All things being equal, every joint in the body is more comfortable and more functional when it is properly aligned. Indeed, the entire body functions better and more comfortably when it's major weight-bearing joints are well aligned, three dimensionally.

Perhaps nothing confirms the biological roots of pain more clearly than a rare condition called congenital insensitivity to pain (CIP). Those born with this condition never develop the nerve cells required to carry sensations of pain to the brain. So of course, without nature's fire alarm, they experience no pain whatsoever. To avoid injuries, they must become hypervigilant of their surroundings but even then, those with this condition are in constant danger of harm.

It's no wonder that pain is often defined as the perception of threat. We need it to alert us to dangers in our environment, internal and external. Without pain, how would you know the coffee is scalding, or that you had just stepped on a nail? Conversely, how do you reconcile the stories about people who suffer dreadful injuries in life-threatening situations and yet, experience absolutely no pain until after the threat had passed? Or what about those who experience phantom limb pain? How can a person feel pain in a body part that doesn't even exist anymore?

If you are wondering how the three-part pain-science model helps explain these different scenarios, you are not alone. The current understanding of CIP suggests that without the necessary nerves to transmit pain to the brain, one's thoughts and feelings about pain matter less than they might otherwise. This could mean that the psychological and emotional components of pain are less than equal partners with the biological component in the pain response equation.

This highlights the fact that local pain factors are subject to how information is managed by the brain. Given its ability to delay pain or cause us to experience phantom sensations, the brain is the control centre for our body's response to pain. Its role is further evident in those instances when people experience pain in the absence of visible signs of injury or irritation.

As one of the last, underexplored frontiers of the human body, the brain is expected to eventually answer the biggest questions about pain. This expectation helps explain how our thoughts and feelings about pain may just be as real, and just as important, as the details of the trigger for that pain.

In 1999, the author of The Mindbody Prescription, Dr. John Sarno, attracted international attention when he proclaimed emotion to be the root cause of most chronic pain. His argument wasn't that pain is purely emotional; it was that most pain begins with a powerful, often overwhelming, emotion. This emotion then causes changes in the body; in particular, changes related to increased muscle tension and reduced blood flow. Beyond certain thresholds, these changes produce pain in local tissues. And yet, by optimizing the position of joints locally and globally, it seems we can minimize how vulnerable these tissues are to pain-producing effects. In further support of the tri-factor model of pain, there is plenty of evidence pointing at how an expectation of success can help tip the scales in favor of overcoming chronic pain.

Currently, so many people experience so little success in eliminating their pain, they get worn out, physically and emotionally. They give up and conclude that their pain is a life sentence. And they resort to doing whatever they can to manage their pain. Chronic pain clinics are literally full of such people.

The good thing about most pain management strategies is that they recognize the multi-faceted character of pain. As a result, they work towards reducing the nervous system load while simultaneously attempting to increase the patient's capacity to cope with that load. The problem with pain management strategies is rarely the strategy itself. The problem often lies in the mindset of the people who struggle to cope with their pain. Too many have completely given up on the hope of ever being pain-free. But whether they believe their pain to be biologically, mentally or emotionally driven, very few people are better off believing that their pain is forever.

How accepting pain as a life sentence works against you. Some years ago, a man in his sixties visited my clinic. He told me he'd been suffering chronic lower back pain, for forty years. From his lack of enthusiasm, I gathered that either his wife or his doctor had made him come to see me. And I remember the last few minutes of that particular session like it was yesterday.

We were finished with the work on the treatment table and I was about to teach him his corrective exercise homework, when he got up and sat on the edge of the table, swearing emphatically! "What did you do to me?", he demanded angrily. I took a moment to collect my thoughts and explained how my work is built upon the idea that misalignment of the skeleton is the underlying cause of most chronic muscle and joint pain. I had found his pelvis to be severely misaligned, had done what I could to straighten it and then used massage techniques, on his lower back and hip muscles, to help them adapt to the straightening.

After a couple seconds of silence that felt like two minutes, he blurted out, "My back pain is gone! If it was that bleeping easy, why didn't someone else do that forty years ago!?!" He stormed out of my treatment room and I never did see him again.

I don't know how long-lived his pain relief was, but I have often wondered how he's doing. I was taken aback by his outburst, but I realized that forty years of pain can build up a lot of frustration and repressed anger. Ironically, his case stands out as a reminder that sometimes, you don't have to explore deep emotional challenges, or even believe a solution is possible, in order to have a successful outcome.

Pain is like misalignment of the skeleton. It changes everything physiologically. It can interfere with your ability to move and be comfortable. It can even impact functions of the body such as heart rate and breathing patterns. And because we're all so different, pain's impacts are unpredictable. But there are some pretty common issues.

Athletes are notorious for continuing to train and compete, in spite of injury. But they're not the only ones who run into trouble with this approach. If you're trying to work around your pain – without simultaneously solving the root cause of your pain – you're likely going to end up with a bigger problem. This is because, if the cause of your pain problem is not corrected, it will, sooner or later, express itself through your body in other ways. It's as if your body is saying: "since my earlier message wasn't understood, I am sending the next message in a different way." Voila! Your lower back pain becomes hip pain. A hamstring strain becomes an Achilles tendon rupture. The tennis elbow becomes a torn rotator cuff. Different problem? Maybe not. Oftentimes your body simply finds a different strategy to get your attention. Disrespect and disregard pain at your own risk.

And wouldn't you know it: we're not good at listening to our own bodies. For proof, just look at the global painkiller market. It's measured in billions of dollars annually. I don't wish anyone to suffer pain unnecessarily; but turning off the fire alarm without putting out the fire is a troublesome strategy. It raises the fundamental issue of perspective. If you adopt the simplistic view that "pain is bad", you are destined to mismanage your problem. Treating it as an inconvenience, that can be ignored with the help of a pill, is to be avoided if at all possible. There is almost always a better way.

You've probably heard something to the effect that the site of physical pain is often not the location of the cause of that pain. I like this this statement because it raises the question, "If lower back pain does not originate in the lower back, then where is it coming from?" The answer usually has something to do with a body part not moving well, resulting in the body making adjustments elsewhere to compensate for that lack of motion. Simply knowing this can be helpful. But to really figure out cause versus effect, you need some kind of assessment.

Unfortunately, testing coordinated movement in the presence of pain is likely to be a measure of pain rather than a test of function. Such assessments can easily be misinterpreted, making it difficult to design an effective treatment plan. That's why assessment/correction of static alignment of the skeleton is one of our first courses of action, when attempting to eliminate chronic pain. Improvement of alignment almost always leads to a lessening of the pain. This paves the way for more accurate assessment and leads to more appropriate and successful therapeutic strategies.

Dr. Eduard Pflüger (1829–1910) was a German physiologist who did as much as anyone to help us understand human neurology, including how pain is expressed in the body. He observed that mild irritation of a nerve tends to result in local signs and symptoms. As the degree of irritation is increased, those signs and symptoms gradually spread to the other side of the body. If the irritation increases beyond a certain level, the signs and symptoms are expressed higher in the body. If irritation becomes intense enough, the brain stem becomes involved to the extent that muscle tone throughout the body is increased. These observations of neurological function are known as Pflüger's Laws. They help us appreciate how the nervous system manages irritation. And because these laws apply whether the irritation is increasing or decreasing, it's reassuring to know that the progressive steps, in this neurological continuum, work just as well in reverse.

To help visualize how your body responds to pain and to signals from your nervous system, I find it helps to think of your ability to cope as being like the storage capacity of your smart phone. Whether it has 16 or 128 Gigabytes, it can only handle so many apps, photos, videos and music files. When it's only half full, you can download just about anything you want. But when near full, you're going to have to make some choices. You either create some room by deleting files or you go without your best friend's latest video. For your phone, it's simply a matter of storage capacity.

That's pretty much how it is for your body, too. Your capacity to deal with nervous system stimulation, in a comfortable, non-painful way, is determined by how much 'storage space' you have to work with. If your 'storage' is only half full, then you have a tremendous amount of wiggle room. You have the capacity to cope with, and adapt to, new stresses in your life. You can sleep in a strange bed, trip over a curb or lift something heavy with no lasting difficulty. However, if your storage space is almost filled with nervous system stimulation, you will have little resilience to the "extra" stresses you encounter in your life.

To continue the analogy, if your 'phone' is almost full of nervous system stimulation, you will be pushed into pain by all kinds of unwanted stressors. Stress at work results in a stomach ache. A quick sprint across the street causes a hamstring strain. An awkward movement triggers pain in the lower back. These negative outcomes are not a function of how young you are, what you eat or how much weight you can lift in the gym. They are a function of how resilient and robust your body is and how overwhelmed your nervous system is. If your 'storage space' is running out, your body is trying to cope with a tremendous amount of physiological stress. Which means you're probably suffering some degree of constant pain.

Our bodies are continually making adjustments. They fight to maintain a steady, healthy state in the face of a dynamic internal/external environment. If your neurological "storage space" is too full, your body has to work overtime, expending effort and energy in an effort to correct the situation. Like the battery in your smartphone, the 'battery' in your body supplies you with a certain amount of energy. If your pain problem is forcing your body into a constant state of emergency, involuntary muscle spasms and perpetual physiological juggling are draining your "battery". Your pain is literally wearing you out.

Hans Selye (1907-1982), an Austrian-born Canadian endocrinologist, developed a theoretical model to explain the human body's response to stress. His model explains how the body responds to challenges in a predictable pattern involving the nervous and hormonal systems. Selye stated that "every stress leaves an indelible scar and the organism pays for its survival after a stressful situation by becoming a little older."

The Pain-Tension Cycle is one of those predictable patterns of how our bodies respond to irritation. It begins when the original problem overwhelms the body's capacity to cope. Whether that problem was caused by injury or by the body trying to adapt to overly repetitive postures or movements, pain begins. That leads to a shortening of the surrounding muscle because that's what they do in an attempt to splint and protect the painful site. This localized muscle tightening reduces the flow of blood and lymphatic fluid which diminishes tissue health. It also decreases joint and tissue mobility. These restrictions in movement promote the development of muscle imbalances. They, in turn, create the prerequisites for subsequent muscle strains, ligament sprains and myofascial trigger points. As they become sources of pain, they lead to further muscle shortening. And so the cycle continues, unless interrupted.

The first step of most rehabilitation processes is to interrupt the Pain-Tension Cycle. The next step involves finding appropriate tools to help support the body unravel all of its layers of compensation, so it can retrace its journey back to a pain-free state.

If there is a secret to getting beyond your pain, it is to increase your capacity to deal with nervous system input and also, decrease the load you need to carry. And whether your pain problem is primarily biological, psychological or emotional, the one common thread is the nervous system. Understanding how this works helps you see how any treatment in such a situation will only be as successful as it is in normalizing the nervous system, both locally and systemically.

Thankfully, both the size of your neurological "storage capacity" and the amount of stuff in it can be changed. Trauma tends to challenge the capacity of your "storage" and over time, can even reduce the size of it. Some therapeutic strategies can lower the volume in your "storage" (how much "stuff" your nervous system has to cope with). Other strategies can increase the size of your "storage" (your capacity to cope with "stuff"). The best strategies, like the Alignment First Protocol, do both. In fact, I believe that daily practice of the protocol is an effective way of minimizing Selye's indelible scars. If I am correct, the protocol can help us age a little more slowly, gracefully and comfortably.

I began this chapter by promising to unravel the mysteries of your chronic issues. I hope you have a better understanding of the purpose of pain, how it's distributed throughout the body and now know some of the things we can do to overcome it. In the next chapter, I'm going to dispel some of the popular misconceptions about lower back pain.

REMEMBER:
Disrespect and disregard pain at your own risk.

CHAPTER 3

What Doesn't Cause Your Pain

*"It ain't what you don't know that gets you in trouble.
It's what you know for sure that just ain't so."*
— MARK TWAIN

As a story-telling species, stories matter to us humans. Stories give us comfort. They define us. And some of our stories stick with us through thick and thin — even when we know they might be more myth than fact. It's just the way we are. However, when these myths and half-truths get in the way of me trying to help you deal with your lower back pain issues, it's time to set the record straight.

If you are like most people, a typical week involves spending 40 hours at work, mostly sitting. There may also be a couple of hours of sitting in your vehicle, and even more hours sitting in front of a TV or computer at home. The actual amount of physical exercise is quite low. Such a lifestyle that combines so much mental/emotional stress with so little physical demand, can be a recipe for dysfunction and disease.

When we look at the exercise many people report doing, we often find that it involves a low level of physical effort. A thirty-minute walk around your neighborhood, a few days a week, is not placing much demand on your body unless you live on the side of a mountain. Most of us got up off the floor and walked when we were about one year of age. Walking around the block may be a healthier alternative to driving around it, but it's not going to result in a stable, well balanced posture. For that, we're going to have to do more than walk a bit.

When I was in elementary school, I was told that future humans would evolve to have very large craniums to hold our ever-increasing brains. Our bodies meanwhile, would resemble stick figures because of the ever-diminishing physical demands of modern life. Part of that hypothetical future seems to be coming true already. That stick figure body, representing physical weakness, is evident all around us, though most of us are thicker not thinner. Our physical weakness, and its accompanying lack of balanced physical demand, is predisposing us to develop muscle imbalances, bony alignment problems and chronic pain.

This predisposition is complicated by our lack of understanding of how the human body works. Unless you're a medical scientist, it's difficult to keep up with the latest research. As modern medicine and its countless branches grows and evolves, the knowledge gap, between scientific fact and public awareness, is growing. This gap fosters the acceptance of incorrect assumptions. It also has negative practical implications.

You've heard the one about not needing to be an electrician in order to operate a light switch? Well, neither do we need to be medical experts in order to perform basic muscle and joint maintenance for ourselves. The ability to help ourselves would, however, be enhanced tremendously if we had a more accurate understanding of what is – and what is not – important to our lower back health and happiness. Popular myths, misunderstandings and old wives' tales often stand in the way of people performing effective back pain self-care.

It's a bit like believing your car is not starting because it is out of gas, when in fact the problem is actually a faulty ignition switch. In this situation, you may never solve the problem, because your belief is obscuring the real issue. Your car is never going to start no matter how much gas you put in the tank. As simple as the actual problem might be, if you're using the wrong solution because you misunderstand the situation, you will fail to solve it. It is pretty much the same for all of life's problems, including your pain issue.

If the root cause of your back pain is somewhere other than your back, as it almost always is, you can manipulate, needle or exercise your back forever and never find relief. And right now, millions of people are suffering chronic back pain, needlessly, simply because they don't understand the nature of their problem. How can you solve a problem you don't understand? Or worse yet, how can you ever resolve something that you believe you understand, when in fact you are holding onto faulty conclusions?

Faulty conclusions can come from well-intentioned friends and family. When they have suffered similar aches and pains, they happily share the solutions that have worked for them. What works for one person should work for others, right?

This kind of thinking reminds me of the 4 Hour series of books by Tim Ferris. This renowned author gets much of his information from self-experimentation. Then he reports on the details of his experiences and wonders aloud if his readers might share similar results. As entertaining as his books are, I remind readers that we cannot draw conclusions that are based only upon the results from one-person case studies. Scientists go to great lengths to separate such subjective, anecdotal reports from data-rich, research studies. I highlight this differential by pointing out that thousands of people have already proven the effectiveness of the Alignment First Protocol, so my trust in the protocol is neither subjective nor anecdotal.

As important as it is to know why you have lower back pain, it is just as important to know what isn't causing your pain. If you think your back pain is inherited, because your mother and grandmother have it, you are unlikely to even try to solve your pain problem. What's the point? If back pain is your destiny, like height and eye color, why bother? That's one point of view.

Here's another. If you don't believe your back pain is inherited, you are more than likely to have a completely different attitude toward your pain. And odds are, you will be quite open to the idea of looking for a solution.

So, come on, let's debunk some of the more persistent and misleading "beliefs" about lower back pain.

1. I'm not 20 anymore.

You'd be surprised how many times I've heard this rationalization from patients in their thirties, forties and even older. It's one of the most overused excuses to explain away lower back pain, even though people of all age suffer its discomfort. I know, because I've helped many teen-agers reorganize their bodies to eliminate their back pain. If there is a time issue related to back pain, it has more to do with how long your skeleton has been misaligned than for how long you've been alive. And yes, your age can be relevant to the conversation, but its degree of importance usually pales in comparison to issues such as bony alignment and movement quality.

Should you be determined to play the age card, keep it up your sleeve until all other options have been explored. That includes finishing this book and giving the protocol a chance to work its magic on your back.

2. I got it from my Mom.

It's human nature to blame our parents' genes for some of our problems. So why should back pain be any different? And in this instance, there's actually a grain of truth to this old wives' tale. Because there are some genetically transmitted health challenges related to the lower back.

The inherited problem that people talk about is scoliosis. As one of the most confusing of spinal issues, Scoliosis refers to lateral curvature of the spine. Its causes are often misunderstood by the medical community, so it is not surprising that it is baffling to the general public as well. When people are told they have scoliosis, they often assume that it is a life sentence. But it is seldom so.

There are three broad types of scoliosis: (1) Congenital, which is caused by bony defects present at birth, (2) Idiopathic, which means "unknown cause", and (3) Scoliosis occurring secondary to some other problem.

A quick Google search confirms that the cause of most scoliosis is unknown. Sources suggest that somewhere between 2-3 percent of the population is affected. My own experience suggests that the vast majority of scoliosis cases are due to secondary causes, such as misalignment of the pelvis. This type of scoliosis probably has little to do with your family tree.

A much less common problem, related to both back pain and genetics, is ankylosing spondylitis. This refers to a chronic inflammatory disease of the spine, in which the bones of the spine (and often the ribcage) fuse together. Statistics suggest that ankylosing spondylitis affects between 0.1 and 0.2% of the population.

So, if only 2-3 percent of the population gets their back pain from their parents via ankylosing spondylitis and scoliosis, where does everyone else get it? Well, from my experience, they often get it from learned behaviour. There is a great deal of literature about how children imitate their parents. Children mimic postures and movement patterns as well as speech patterns and mannerisms. They thereby inherit their parents' dysfunctional posture and movement patterns, and as a result, they often end up with the same chronic pain problems as well. So, parents, please pay attention and be cognizant of your posture. Or as my mother would say, stand up straight!

3. I've got one leg shorter than the other.

You probably do have one leg shorter than the other. But to have significant differences in the length of the long bones of your legs, is rare. It is way more common to have a pelvis that isn't perfectly "square". Indeed, some years ago, I was treating an athlete in a training room, with a medical doctor present. The athlete had an alignment problem with his pelvis and it was having a direct, causative effect on his acutely sore lower back. I chatted with the doctor while I worked, explaining that I was helping the athlete return his pelvis to a more neutral position. Somewhat surprised by my comments, the doctor told me that such a thing was not possible. He was sure that there is no significant amount of independent movement between the different pelvic bones.

Well! I think you can imagine how awkward the conversation became. Because I know for a fact that the sacrum and both iliums (two of the bones that form the pelvis) move independently of one another. A significant percentage of my patients need help correcting the misalignments between these bones. So, if you take away nothing else from this book, please understand that most chronic lower back pain problems are avoidable; and that a large percentage of those problems stem, at least in part, from a pelvic alignment problem.

Back to the leg length issue. Our thigh bones attach to our pelvic bones via the hip joint. If one side of the pelvis (the ilium) rotates forward or back, relative to the other side of the pelvis and stays there, you will be the unwitting owner of both a crooked pelvis and a functional leg length difference. It's called functional, as opposed to structural, because the difference in leg length is due to the way in which your body is organized. It's not due to an actual bony difference. The good news is that straightening your pelvis will either eradicate the leg length differential, or it will get you one step closer to eliminating it. Either way, you'll be getting closer to enjoying a happier lower back.

4. I sit all day.

According to some media reports, "sitting is the new smoking". Maybe I'm missing something here, but I just don't see that in my practice. Granted, doing anything for hours, without significant change of position or demand, is less than ideal. But when I hear anti-sitting experts saying things that run counter to what I am seeing in my clinic, I have to speak up.

They say that because you are sitting all day, your body adaptively shortens your hip flexor muscles. Then, when you stand up at the end of the day, you are still somewhat hip flexed. Their argument is consistent with how the soft tissues of the body adapts to any constantly repeated posture or activity. And I do believe that a chronically hip flexed posture leads to unnecessarily tight hips and lower back hyperextension. However, in spite of society's epidemic of sitting, I see far more cases of back and hip pain involving hips that are hyperextended rather than hyperflexed.

Why does this disparity exist? My interpretation is that the biggest obstacle to establishing neutral pelvic and hip positioning is actually a weakness, or if you prefer, an overall deconditioning of the muscles in the area. It is not chronic hip flexor shortening. Even when I see people who have their pelvis rotated too far forward, a positional problem that should be consistent with hyperflexed hips, I see hyperextended hips far more often than hyperflexed ones. I agree that any position held for hours on end and repeated day after day, is an unhealthy way to live.

But I do not agree that millions of people are walking around with chronic lower back pain because of shortened hip flexor muscles caused by our culture of sitting. Overall weakness is a much bigger problem than short hip flexors.

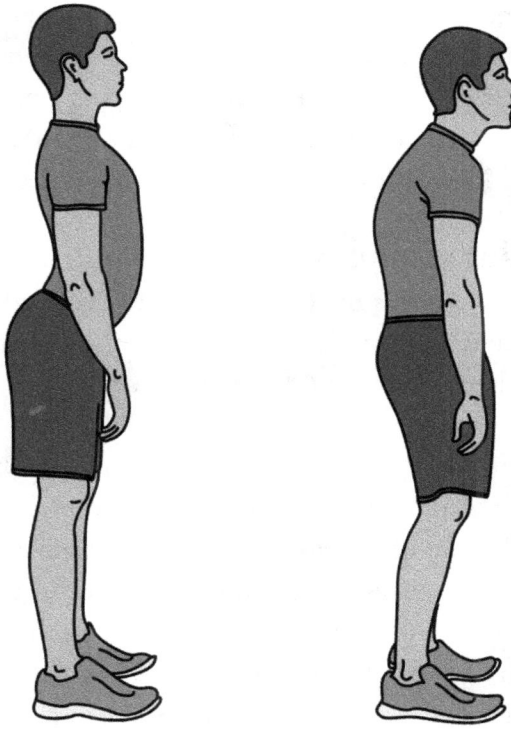

Hyperflexed Hips and Hyperextended Hips

5. My abs are weak.

This is another example of a myth that has some truth to it. Broadly speaking, since your abs connect your ribcage to your pelvis, these muscles do need to be strong enough to allow your ribcage and pelvis to align vertically. These core muscles also need the strength to coordinate your upper and lower body for whole body movements. So, certainly, if your abdominal muscles are weak, they can contribute to chronic lower back pain.

However, to suggest that chronic back pain can be solved with a regimen of ab crunches, is a dangerous half-truth. I have worked with too many people who could perform hundreds of abdominal crunches, but who still suffered from lower back pain.

If your lower back muscles are chronically contracted and painful, tightening your abs to an equally shortened state is not going to be beneficial. What ends up happening is a tightening and compression of every structure in your lower spine. This approach puts your spine in a vise and probably sets you on a fast track for a disc herniation, with your next stop being lower back surgery. Not a good strategy, that.

6. "My gluteus medius won't fire."

Blaming the lowly gluteus medius muscle for lower back pain is something that's been rather popular for the last few years. How this become such a trend I do not know, but I can't wait for this one to ride off into the sunset.

Sometimes this muscle won't activate at the proper time or with the proper intensity. And though this problem could be the primary cause of chronic back pain, in the vast majority of cases that I have seen, an inhibited gluteus medius is more of an effect, than a cause.

It's pretty much a matter of how misalignment impairs neuromuscular function. If you test your gluteus medius when your pelvis is misaligned and then, test it again, *after* the positional problem has been corrected, the muscle consistently and reliably shows improved function. It is a natural result of neutral positioning. And as you might imagine, if you try to strengthen this muscle without first re-establishing proper pelvic alignment, the process will be inefficient at best. At worst, it may not work at all.

Here's a dietary analogy that may give you some perspective on the skeletal/muscular continuum. When trying to lose weight, people often worry about getting the right amount of protein, fats and carbohydrates in their diet. But what they should really be concerned about is overeating. No amount of nutrient manipulation will help you lose weight if you do not indulge in portion control. In this analogy, portion control takes precedence over macro nutrient ratio.

To solve your lower back pain puzzle, skeletal alignment takes precedence over muscular function. Why? It just does. There is no reason to indulge in movement re-education, if your skeleton is too compromised to even get into the proper starting position. You will be much more successful in relieving your lower back pain if you accept that structural issues always take precedence over the soft tissue ones. And getting that priority right will make all the difference between success and failure.

That's pretty much it for the most common examples of what isn't causing your lower back pain. Let's now move on to the six issues that are more important for lower back health and happiness.

REMEMBER:

As important as it is to know why you have lower back pain, it is just as important to know what isn't causing your pain.

If there is a time issue related to back pain, it has more to do with how long your skeleton has been misaligned than for how long you've been alive.

CHAPTER 4

Painful Principles

"Malalignment of the pelvis, spine and extremities remains one of the frontiers of medicine, unrecognized as a cause of over 50% of back and limb pain."
— DR. WOLFGANG SCHAMBERGER MD.

In this chapter, we transition from myths and misconceptions to actual problems that plague our bodies and cause our backs so much pain. Here follows an explanation of the six issues most likely to cause lower back pain. Understand them and you might just get the Pareto Principle working for you.

The 80/20 Rule, also known as the Pareto Principle, states that 80 percent of your results come from 20 percent of your efforts. The principle applies to every subject in every field of endeavour and its benefits are delightful: if you can determine the issues that constitute the critical 20 percent, you'll have discovered the key to efficiency. This book aims to help you understand the key information relevant to lower back pain, so you can apply the principle and enjoy its benefits. (I hope this sounds as good to you as it does to me.)

1. Alignment (or the lack of it)

How can lower back pain be the single most common and expensive chronic pain problem in North America? How can it cost us billions of dollars in the form of lost wages, healthcare expenses and productivity losses? Why is it such a common problem? The answer is the same for all three questions: the vast majority of people are posturally asymmetrical. How your body structure is organized is a key determinant of whether or not you will develop muscle pain and/or joint pain.

It would be wonderful if everyone had a body that assumed a perfectly neutral posture. Because when bony alignment is perfectly arranged, all the major weight-bearing joints work together. This harmony minimizes the muscular effort required to oppose gravity and to move the body in a coordinated manner. All things being equal, such a body is healthier, more functional and more comfortable than with any other posture.

Our muscles and their tendons perform like guy wires. They're designed to support our bones against the pull of gravity. When our joints are stacked, one on top of the other, they maximize the bony support and minimize the effort our muscles expend to hold us upright. This stacking concept brings to mind a vision of the Eiffel Tower and how it differs from the Leaning Tower of Pisa. Imagine them side by side and you get to see a good and a bad posture. One looks strong and stable. The other appears to defy gravity. They're both beautiful, but this is not about aesthetics; it's about function and comfort. Which begs the question: which one has chronic back pain? Not the one in France.

When I consider how widespread postural asymmetry is, I am surprised that more people don't suffer from chronic pain. Those who are chronically challenged are usually doubly afflicted. Their alignment problems are significant enough to be aggravated by additional challenges. As for those of us who are not suffering ongoing pain, our alignment issues are either of a lesser degree or our nervous systems are not yet overwhelmed. More often than not, our pain-free status is a result of both conditions being mild enough to not set off any alarms.

In my clinic, I see some people with noticeably distorted postures who have no perception of their alignment problem; only an awareness of their pain. Others are cognizant of their alignment problems because they've looked in the mirror or it's been drawn to their attention; but they don't suffer any pain. Both situations are a testament to the incredible ability of the human body to cope with stress. But just because the body can compensate and, in the latter case, not complain with pain, people should not ignore their obvious asymmetries. The assumption that there is no problem because there is no pain is a flawed interpretation.

Maybe you've had a seamstress put a shoulder pad in your jacket to hide a low shoulder. Maybe your tailor hems one pant leg a little shorter than the other. It's too easy to treat these imbalances as aesthetic inconveniences and hide them with clever tailoring. But here's the thing: they're clear evidence of tension imbalances. They usually cause accelerated wear and tear on joint structures. Which means they are going to become sources of pain, sooner or later.

As I like to say, the good news about most alignment issues is that they are functional not structural. That means they can be corrected. We can teach the body how to become better aligned. And in the process, we can rebuild a foundation that restores healthy mobility, improves muscle function and strengthens the nervous system. This more neutral posture may not guarantee the end of pain, but it will create an environment where pain-free is actually possible.

Of all the misalignment issues, it's been my experience that the most common cause of lower back pain is when the top and bottom of the pelvis are no longer parallel with the ground. This condition often leads to people complaining that one of their legs is shorter than the other. And as mentioned earlier, such leg length discrepancies are usually "functional" not "structural". In other words, they are caused by a soft tissue tension imbalance. They are not a result of an actual difference in the length of the bones of the legs.

I hasten to add that those who must wear an orthotic to compensate for the short leg are right to do so, when there is a true bony difference. But when the cause of their leg-length differential is a soft tissue imbalance, an insert in one's shoe is no solution at all. It might provide some temporary relief but, unfortunately, it prevents you from actually solving the real problem. To do that, it's best to seek out the proper corrective strategy. One that releases the shortened soft tissues in the pelvis/hip/thigh of the "shorter leg". It works for most people by eliminating their symptoms.

Not surprisingly, the second most common cause of alignment related, lower back pain is also in the pelvic area. The problem arises when the entire pelvis has rotated either too far forward, or too far back.

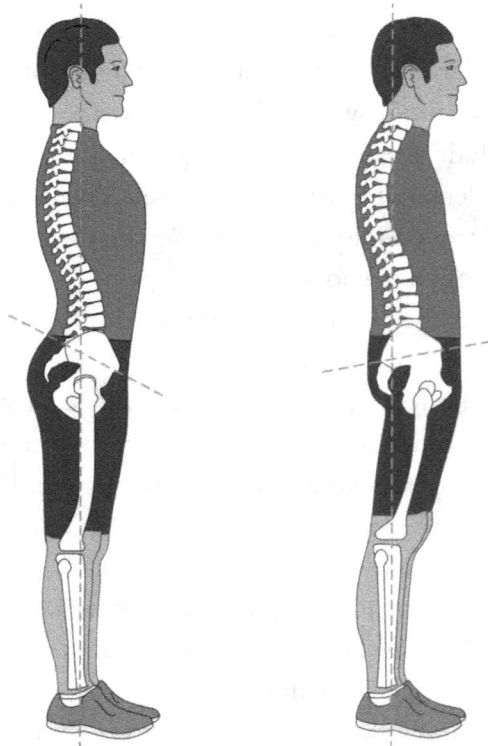

Hyperlordotic Posture and Hyperkyphotic Posture

Certain muscle imbalances in the lower back, abdomen, hips and thighs can cause excessive rotation of the pelvis. When the rotation is too far forward, as shown in the above left figure, it will often occur with excessive curvature in the lumbar spine. This curvature compresses the facet joints, which are the small posterior joints between each vertebra in your spine. Over time, this sort of spinal compression leads to painful irritation which brings on degenerative changes, ranging from osteoarthritis to degenerative disc disease.

Alternately, if the rotation is too far back, as shown in the above right figure, it often occurs with insufficient curvature of the spine. This causes instability, which is something the body hates. So, it responds in one of two ways. It will either attempt to splint the spine with muscle spasm. Or, it will compensate by forcing the entire pelvis forward (tucking your tailbone under and walking down the street by leading with your belt buckle).

When the pelvis is pushed forward like this, out in front of the knees and shoulders, a curve will be restored to the lower back. This is called having your hips extended. And it results in a posture known as a sway back. But now, since the overall alignment of the body, relative to gravity, has been so completely altered, this compensation is almost always followed by others. The next most notable compensation being an exaggerated upper back curvature and head-forward posture. It's called hyperkyphosis which, to me, sounds like an appropriate name for the high cost the body is paying to re-create that curve in the lower back. When all these compensations are stacked on top of each other, the body is forced to struggle to stay upright against the pull of gravity. Is it any wonder people with this sort of posture are so chronically tired and sore?

Look at the tilt of the shoulders in the following figure and you will see the third most common cause of lower back pain. When shoulders are in such different positions relative to one another, you know there's a problem. It often causes pain in three locations: the upper back, the neck and the lower back. For those with a shoulder height differential of an inch or more, they will usually complain of lower back pain on the same side as their "low shoulder". Such obvious shoulder height differentials are often accompanied by pelvic alignment problems as well.

Should pelvic alignment not be problematic in such a case, relief for the lower back can often be found by gently stretching the soft tissues of the lower back and torso. Since they are responsible for the depression of the "low shoulder" and the resulting compression of the spine, their release often gives relief from pain.

The key concept to keep in mind is that joint misalignment causes instability. Since the body will do whatever it can to reacquire stability, its stabilization strategy is to use muscle spasm as a sort of muscular corset. If uncorrected, this type of muscular compensation creates muscle fatigue, then irritation, followed by further muscle shortening as a self defense mechanism. Sound familiar?

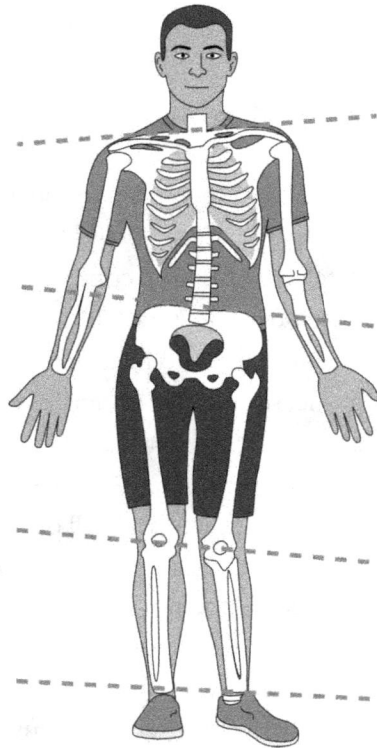

Wedge Posture

This is how the Pain-Tension Cycle, discussed in Chapter 2, is born. When layers of different muscular compensations don't add enough stability, interesting postures and movement patterns begin to appear. None of them are comfortable, and none are healthy. Such a poor base of support gives rise to the expression "It's like trying to shoot a cannon out of a canoe". Often heard in the weight room, it's meant to be amusing. But the postural pattern of feet pointed out like a duck, knees coming together and a crooked pelvis on top of it all, is no laughing matter. It's unstable, dysfunctional and painful.

2. Muscle Balance (or the lack of it)

The kissing cousin of misalignment is muscle imbalance. Imbalance exists when one muscle prevents another from remaining at its normal resting length. Imbalance also occurs when a muscle prevents the joint it crosses from moving through its full range of motion.

These 'cousins' are interesting in that they effect each other differently. On the one hand, traumatic misalignment usually creates a muscle imbalance. But on the other, the insidious development of muscle imbalance may or may not result in misalignment. When it does, it's pretty obvious.

For instance, the most recognizable example of how muscle imbalance affects the human body is stereotypically called the "little old lady" posture. The Hunchback of Notre Dame also contributed some fame to the condition. More formally known as hyperkyphosis, it occurs when the muscles in the front of the neck and torso shorten so much that the entire spine flexes forward. The muscles that should oppose this forward flexion are either pathologically weakened or they just get overpowered.

Most people with a hyperkyphotic posture suffer from chronic back and neck pain, along with headaches. Because of the severity of their chronic symptoms, people in this situation commonly receive professional therapy treatments to manage their pain. But if that therapy is applied to the back or to the back of the neck, it is doomed to failure. Here's why.

The reason their back and neck muscles are so sore is because they are being overstretched by the pull of muscles, in the front of the body. When therapies are aimed at relaxing the painful back and neck muscles, all they do is allow them to lengthen even further. This lengthening will almost always make the situation worse, not better. For treatment to succeed, it must involve an attempt to relax and lengthen the shortened muscles in the front of the body, since they're the ones that are forcing the spine forward. The abdominal and chest muscles are the usual targets for this strategy.

The key principle here is one touched on earlier. Your bones are the tent poles of your body. And your muscles and tendons are guy wires that hold the whole structure up, off the ground. When your guy wires are not equal in terms of length, flexibility or strength, you get muscle imbalance. If severe enough, such imbalances lead to misalignment of the skeleton and a decrease in healthy physical function. You may very well not experience any pain, but that's only because your body is able to compensate.

Keep in mind that such compensations are supposed to be temporary. Your body is buying you time until you can return to "normal". But if you're like most of us, you are walking around with a number of other muscular compensations. They've become part of your regular repertoire of function. But there is a cost to these compensations. They're quite inefficient, so once the body's first attempt at compensation fatigues, it throws a second layer of compensation at the problem. Over time, these issues build up like dust bunnies under the bed, unobserved and unwanted. In most cases, we are not even aware of them. So, we do nothing as they accumulate. In response, our body begins to "get older" and more dysfunctional, regardless of our actual age.

Before moving onto muscle tightness, I should add that other, less obvious, muscle imbalances can occur almost anywhere in the body and they can and will affect anyone at any age.

One very common complaint that I've heard over the years, is how tight a certain muscle is and that no matter how long or how frequently it is stretched, the muscle simply will not relax. The culprits are commonly the hamstrings and the upper back. The explanation for this problem is deceptively simple. The tight muscle in question will not stretch, despite your best efforts, because it is already stretched.

The urge to stretch a tight muscle is a human instinct. It's almost an automatic response. But in this instance, stretching tight muscles does more harm than good. Muscles get tight whenever they are not at their normal resting length. However, a muscle can deviate from its normal resting length by being either shorter or longer than it should be, when at rest. The general rule is that a muscle that is too short should be stretched, but a muscle that is already too long will not benefit from being stretched.

When athletes have shortened quads, they often fall prey to the above situation regarding their hamstrings. Their actual problem is chronically shortened quadriceps, compared to their hamstrings. But their experience of it – their sense of it, if you like - is that their hamstrings feel really tight. But stretching them is not going to help. The solution almost always depends upon the shortened quadriceps being stretched. Doing so reduces the stretch tension on the hamstrings. I don't want to make that process sound too easy because, when the hamstrings have been overstretched for years, it is often necessary for these muscles to be retrained. This can be accomplished with strengthening exercises that coax them back towards their normal resting length and into a more balanced relationship with the quads.

An interesting piece of this particular puzzle occurs when the quad/hip flexor group of muscles is stretched. It commonly results in a pelvic position improvement that has a powerful, normalizing influence on the quadriceps, the hamstrings and on the critically important hip and core muscles as well.

The word 'insidious' comes to mind whenever I discuss chronic conditions in the absence of an obvious injury. Most chronic pain arises from the gradual development of muscle imbalances. For example, when the lower back muscles, the quadriceps and the hip flexors are too short, they overpower the weaker abdominals, glutes and hamstrings. The facet joints of the lower back get hyperextended and compressed, which leads to a common positional problem. The most obvious sign of this posture being an overly large curve in the lower back, called hyperlordosis.

If muscle imbalances are severe enough and if the resulting positional problem persists long enough, you will eventually experience some degree of chronic lower back pain. But since the conditions evolve so gradually, the problem remains outside of your conscious awareness. When the pain finally does strike, the standard response is to wonder "what's wrong with my back? I didn't do anything to it". It's so frustrating and baffling, most sufferers can't help but wonder what dark forces have conspired to bring about this mysterious problem. They probably have no idea that the process that caused their pain has been evolving for years, maybe decades.

Relief may be a long and slow process. Or it may be delightfully promising from the outset, as it was for the following patient. She's a Masters track and field athlete who was experiencing chronic hip/thigh and back pain. Here's an email she sent, a few days after her first session:

"Have your ears been burning? I feel fantastic, the best I have felt in years. I believe it is thanks to your session. I have consistently completed the exercises since last Sunday, once each day. I wanted to experience the exercises along with three workout and weight training sessions.

"I noticed a difference on the Friday after our session. We often practice certain drills over hurdles and, don't laugh, but I felt taller! These types of drills help with mobility and flexibility. I am usually in pain and complaining as I do the drills. I have completed the drills twice and I feel great going over the hurdles. I have more range of motion doing the drills . . . I'm sure you know what I mean.

"As for running, I notice that I'm running without that tentative feeling, like I'm cautious with each stride. The last part of the warm up involves five strides. My first stride is usually the worst. I usually feel stiff and I notice pain in my knees and tension in my shoulders. If someone were watching me warm up they would be surprised to know I'm a sprinter! Yikes. I immediately noticed a difference this past week in my strides. They are faster and virtually pain-free! The pain I suffer in my lower back is a dull pain. It is always present. Usually after the workout on the way home . . . with the heated seats on high to prevent seizing up . . . I feel the tension and pain especially on the right side of my lower back and hip. After this week the pain is noticeably less."

The changes she describes occurred during the first week of her exposure to the Alignment First Protocol. Her story also illustrates that even elite athletes develop muscle imbalances. Rare is the person who consistently applies enough balanced physical demand on their body to maintain healthy muscle balance and posture. The fact that these imbalances are all around us is, I believe, the single biggest reason physical asymmetry has come to be accepted as "normal".

Now let's look at how imbalance can lead to mobility problems which can vary from excessive range of movement to too little.

3. Mobility (or the lack of it)

Essentially, mobility is how far you can move a joint, without external influence. Every joint in the body has a range of motion that is considered to be "normal". There are such things as too much and, conversely, too little range of motion.

For better or worse, the issue of too little range of motion has historically been addressed with stretching. But for quite some time now, prominent members of the rehabilitation community have been banging the drum about the inefficiency of stretching. In certain situations, I find myself agreeing with them, wholeheartedly. Many cases of glaring mobility restriction, for example, are primarily caused by the body reacting to a lack of stability. In these cases, it is easy to show how increasing stability of the trunk, via contraction of core muscles, can quickly increase the range of motion in a hip that was previously restricted. It is also immediately clear, that you cannot stretch this kind of tightness away.

The best route past a stability-caused restriction is to reorganize the body positionally, and then stabilize the improvements. If it is appropriate to use some exercises that are considered to be stretches to reorganize the body positionally, so be it. But bear in mind that it is the neutral positioning that triggers soft tissue and nervous system improvements, not the "stretching" of the muscles. My comments are not an indictment against stretching. I merely caution that stretching, like any other tool, is appropriate some of the time. And sometimes it's not.

There is a relatively common mobility problem that I was strangely unaware of, until a few years ago. It was drawn to my attention by Evan Osar, an expert on assessment, corrective exercise and integrative movement. He pointed out how the body compensates for a lack of mobility in the torso, by creating extra mobility in the spine, right below the ribcage. This dysfunctional and often painful hinging cannot be remedied by any treatment at the site of pain. Neither can you reliably eliminate the hypermobility at the site of pain, until after you have increased the mobility of the ribcage. This is a beautiful and clear illustration of the hierarchical nature of the rehab process. Until you take care of Job One, do not pass Go and do not collect 200 dollars.

Your body will often reveal your Achilles Heel (vulnerable spot) via hypermobility. It usually does this in response to a lack of mobility elsewhere. The most recognized example of this phenomenon is when the lower back hyperextends, at least partially, due to excessive shortening of the hip flexor muscles. I say "at least partially" because a strong and stable lower back will not necessarily be pulled into hyperextension in this way. However, as a matter of simple mechanics, two things can be expected when the hip flexors are too short. Either the lower back becomes hyperextended or the hips become hyperflexed. In this tug of war, these are the only real possibilities.

The human body is elegantly designed for movement. A balanced body is so efficient, it moves in a biomechanically correct and almost effortless manner. And yet, an unbalanced body can move surprisingly well, too. It just has to get creative and find ways to move in spite of mobility restrictions. And though such a body may not be ideal, you can live with it if you don't mind the accelerated wear and tear and "a little" chronic pain. That's one option. My preferred option is for you to resolve your glaring alignment problems. Doing so can ensure that you reacquire full range of motion in all of your major weightbearing joints. Better yet, it will move you along the path towards becoming pain-free.

And now, let's shift focus away from range of movement, to the quality of your movement.

4. Stability (or the lack of it)

A properly organized body is a marvellous platform designed to deliver stability. For instance, when your legs and joints fold smoothly into a squatting position, your bones and soft tissues collaborate elegantly to hold the weight of your body, making the squat a comfortable, resting position. Such interplays of bones, joints and muscles can lead us into pain or deliver us from its grasp.

Some people would have you believe that hypermobility (the ability to move beyond what is considered "normal" range of motion at any given joint) is a major cause of pain. And yet, a quick search on YouTube shows many examples of people who have incredible mobility plus, the strength and coordination to control that mobility. We've touched on the pain caused by the misalignment and imbalance "cousins". And we've considered their impact on our health. Let's now look at how the cousins can also create weakness and instability, via muscle inhibition. As to whether the observed "weaknesses" are true physiological weaknesses, or simply temporary losses of motor control, they're moot points for now.

One type of muscle inhibition is called reciprocal inhibition. This occurs when muscles on one side of a joint relax and lengthen to accommodate the muscle shortening, on the other side. All joints are controlled by two opposing sets of muscles that work together, in a coordinated manner, to produce smooth movement at the joint. When one of the paired muscles shortens, a trick of the nervous system triggers a degree of de-activation, allowing for controlled lengthening of the opposing muscle. Like a sound system, when the "volume" on the one muscle is turned up, the "volume" on the other is turned down.

This feature of the nervous system becomes problematic, however, when the controls get "stuck". As you might expect, this little hitch is caused by chronic muscle imbalances and misaligned joints. It's difficult to be strong and stable when, on a whim, your nervous system can turn your muscle controls "down" or even, turn them "off". When you're standing still, you may very well have the necessary strength to provide an acceptable amount of stability. But when you go to move, that increase in demand for stability may exceed your ability to deliver. Such an inability to meet your body's strength and stability demands will lead to problems. You will become susceptible to the development of dysfunctional compensation patterns of stabilization and movement. Whether they lead to chronic pain or recurring injury, these issues are going to leave you in a bad place. Essentially, you'll become an accident waiting to happen.

When Gray Cook, a prominent physiotherapist, and Mike Boyle, a preeminent strength and conditioning coach, came up with the Joint by Joint Concept, they captured everyone's attention. (Well, everyone involved in physiological science, practice and rehabilitation, that is.) Their concept described a whole new way of looking at the body that changed just about everything.

This model states that mechanically speaking, the body is a system of alternating stable and mobile segments. The mobile segments gain leverage from the stable segments to effectively produce force. Like *yin and yang,* the concept is simple, brilliant and true. Its relevance to this discussion of stability (or the lack of it) is this: when joints that are supposed to be stable become hypermobile, you lose stability. And you either have, or are on your way to, a chronic pain situation. In this instance, I am referring to the lower back and pelvis. The problems arise because the body is poorly organized positionally, functionally or both.

And then there's an interesting flip side to the model. The stable and mobile segments in the body can actually get reversed. They trade places. Instead of your lower back and pelvis being stable, they respond to your rigid torso and "tight" hips by becoming more mobile than they should be. Your body is beginning to overcompensate and that is never a good thing. A much better strategy is to train your body to be functionally consistent with the Joint by Joint Concept. This will keep you pointed in the right direction. Just as your socks should go on before your shoes, there is a proper way for the body to be organized. Recognize and respect that fact and you'll get more than a fighting chance to become pain-free.

5. Stress (and Your Nervous System)

Hans Selye was an Austrian-born Canadian endocrinologist who developed a theoretical model to explain the human body's response to stress. He called it the General Adaptation Syndrome, later renaming it the Stress Response. His model explains how the body responds to challenge. It's a predictable pattern that involves both the nervous and hormonal systems.

> *"Every stress leaves an indelible scar, and the organism pays for its survival after a stressful situation by becoming a little older".*
> — HANS SELYE (1907-1982)

Dr. Selye outlined three distinct phases of the Stress Response:

1. Alarm Stage
2. Resistance Stage
3. Exhaustion Stage

He warns that by the time you have reached the Exhaustion Stage of the Stress Response, the body has used up most of its resources in trying to cope with stress. Over time, its coping ability is diminished. This decrease can be gradual or abrupt. Meanwhile, your immune system also gets dragged into the fray where it is also likely to become exhausted.

People with chronic pain commonly find themselves living within the Exhaustion Stage of the Stress Response. They're overwhelmed and exhausted, both physically and emotionally. And as noted in Chapter 3, when discussing genetic contributions to the chronic pain puzzle, if you happen to have inherited a nervous system with lower pain tolerance, your vulnerability to finding yourself down and out in the Exhaustion Stage of the Stress Response is that much greater.

Remember that nothing done to your lower back will make you feel better if your entire nervous system is overwhelmed. It has its limits and when you overload it, you often need appropriate care to calm the entire nervous system. And that's in addition to cracking the code on the root cause of your chronic pain problem.

6. Misunderstanding (and Expectation)

Tiger Woods is a fine golfer. Some say he's the greatest of his generation and others consider him to be the greatest golfer of all time. Unfortunately, he is showing signs of being "broken". It's an understatement to say he has had some injury problems. Better to pointedly ask, why has he had *so many* injuries? Opinions vary but they typically cite his aggressive swing and his strength training. Many say he's too muscular to have a healthy back as a golfer. But I disagree with these comments.

To me, his efforts to get ever stronger and create a new golf swing every couple of years is a classic example of misunderstanding the problem. By definition such misunderstanding results in misdirected efforts. I believe he has skeletal misalignment issues. In spite of everything he does for his athletic conditioning and his exceptional sport-specific skills, Tiger's back is proving to be his Achilles heel. And I fear his failure to understand and effectively correct the underlying misalignment will hasten the premature end of his illustrious career.

We've all seen it happen before. I'm not talking about acute career ending injuries, like Joe Theismann's broken leg or Michael Irvin's fractured spine. I'm referring to superstars who were plagued by one injury after another, like Bill Walton (one of the NBA's best centres of all time) and Tracy McGrady (one of the highest NBA scorers in a single game). Misunderstanding of the root causes of their issues helped end their careers, prematurely.

I encountered an athlete who would experience such a shortened career, back in 1991. That's when I met Jason Herter, in Victoria, during training camp for the Vancouver Canucks Hockey Club. Jason had been the first-round pick of the Canucks in the 1989 Entry Draft and the number 8 draft choice overall in the NHL that year. Midway through his freshman year at the University of North Dakota, he had been ranked as the top player available for the 1989 NHL Entry Draft. That year, he also set assist and point records for a freshman defenceman at North Dakota.

Jason had an incredibly bright future ahead of him. However, he played only one NHL game in his entire career. He bounced around the IHL, AHL and German Ice Hockey League for ten years. The official story is that Jason's career was hampered by "chronic groin problems". But that's just a classic case of "describing the water". Pelvic alignment problems were the primary reason Jason never fulfilled his potential to be an NHL All-Star.

I know this because when I began working with Jason, he was struggling with recurring, acute lower abdominal strains, commonly called a sports hernia. I knew it was caused by the misalignment of his pelvis but back then, I didn't know what to do about it. Given how common sports hernias were at that time, most other practitioners didn't seem to know how to correct the problem either. It was exasperating. Indeed, the frustration I experienced while working with Jason, has since directed the path of my development as a therapist. Amongst many other things, I now know how to effectively treat a misaligned pelvis.

Assessment and treatment are like detective work. If you can find the problem and trace it back to the cause, you can usually devise a solution. You know muscle imbalances lead to dysfunctional positioning. You know dysfunction leads to joint irritation and pain. Those two "knowns" dramatically increase the odds of achieving success in treatment. And yes, there are those occasional problems with mysterious causes. Then it's a real challenge to come up with a plan of action that you can confidently pursue. In such cases, your only hope is that the forces of good can somehow overcome the forces of evil, that have obviously descended upon you in error.

And yes, I know. Without an action-based solution to focus on, you are likely to resort to pain medication as your primary therapeutic tool. But I urge patience, diligence and determination. Because when you understand the true source of the problem, you will likely find the necessary motivation to pursue a logical strategy aimed at eliminating the problem for good. A well thought out treatment plan, at the very least, implies a resolution of the problem is possible and maybe, even within sight. This helps create an expectation of success. And an expectation of success has been proven to greatly enhance the possibility of success in any endeavor.

That being said, I shake my head in dismay at human nature. It seems determined to find shortcuts around long-term, daily regimens that have proven to be beneficial. I think you would be astounded at how often I've heard a version of the following: "I was doing the exercises and feeling great, so I gradually stopped doing them, and now the pain is back."

Like many of my peers, I struggle to convince patients that treatment for pain relief is a process. That means the course of action can be ongoing for quite some time. For sure, some people enjoy great results after only two or three clinic visits. Many sense improvement after the first few weeks of consistently following their corrective exercise prescription. But it can take months, and even years, to overcome the complex imbalances and compensations they've accumulated. A few weeks of getting good at the exercises cannot erase decades of bad alignment and movement habits. Yet those exercises can launch a process of improvement that many have called magical. And yes, I know, who else but a therapist would dare suggest that a daily regimen can be magic. But that's just it. It almost is.

Without pain meds and without complicated medical procedures, a routine of daily practice, for a year or more, usually results in a degree of mastery of a process that earns you the right to "take some time off", without your pain reminding you to get back to it. Most people who commit to mastering these exercises to this degree, usually get respite from big muscle imbalances, alignment problems and chronic pain.

Now that you have an insight on the six issues most likely to cause chronic back pain, we are going to move on and talk about the effects of those problems.

REMEMBER:

As I like to say, the good news about most alignment issues is that they are functional not structural. That means they can be corrected.

This more neutral posture may not guarantee the end of pain, but it will create an environment where pain-free is actually possible.

CHAPTER 5
Painful Parts

"Divide each difficulty into as many parts as is feasible and necessary to resolve it."
— RENE DESCARTES

This chapter talks about your spine, vertebrae and discs and how your body abuses them with its misalignments, imbalances and compensations. Since your back is where most of your postural problems are expressed, it helps to understand what the important parts are, why they hurt and how you can make them better.

But first, let's take a brief aside to highlight some misconceptions that reside in patients' comments, when talking about their backs. Many describe their issues by saying something similar to: "I bent over to pick up a towel, when my back went out" or, "I must have slept funny because I woke up with back pain". I still don't know what "sleeping funny" actually looks like, but that statement always makes me smile. And please, can someone tell me where your back goes, when it "goes out"? What actually happens in such cases?

The answer lies within the anatomy of your spine. You know it's segmented and that each vertebra in the spine connects with its neighboring vertebrae. You may not know that these joints are called 'facet joints'. (Now you do.) Or that there are four facet joints on each vertebra, two that articulate (form a joint) with the vertebra above and two that articulate with the vertebra below. This is how all the bones in your spine link up with each other.

When you flex your spine (bend forward), the facet joints open (pull apart). When you extend your spine (bend backward), the facet joints close (get closer together). Most back pain is caused when one or more of these facet joints fails to move properly. Specifically, facet joints can end up getting stuck open or closed. Sometimes they're not completely stuck, but nevertheless they're unable to move smoothly through a full range of motion.

When a facet joint is stuck closed, or unable to open as far as you are asking it to, you will likely experience pain when you try to flex your spine forward. The same is true for a facet joint that is stuck open. It'll be painful when you extend your spine backwards.

When dealing with this type of joint dysfunction, it helps to realize that the joint is not dislocated. It has not gone "out" of whack. The joint is still operating within its normal range of motion; it's just not moving properly. The resolution of this problem is not about putting the joint back where it belongs. Resolution is about helping it move like it is supposed to. Correcting this type of dysfunction is the foundation for classic chiropractic and osteopathic care.

Many structural alignment problems will leave you at risk of developing facet joint dysfunction. For example, a pelvis that is higher on one side than the other, will cause the spine to bend a little to the side and rotate. The facet joints, on the side that the spine is rotating towards, will be closed more than those on the opposite side. If this condition is allowed to persist for years, the soft tissues on that side of the spine adapt and gradually shorten to reflect this more "closed" positioning. If you then ask those tissues, that have gradually shortened, to suddenly lengthen more fully than they are able to, you may experience an overstretch injury (muscle strain). That strain will then cause those muscles to shorten even further, as the body endeavours to protect itself from injury.

This is an example of muscular compensation. It's how the body increases stability. Unfortunately, it's almost always at the cost of placing increased mechanical pressure on the joint. This excess pressure leads to tissue irritation. That causes muscle contraction which leads to yet more joint pressure. Eventually, that simple muscular compensation can develop into a self-perpetuating, downward spiral of pain and dysfunction.

As time passes, the soft tissues around the joint become accustomed to their shortened state. If it goes on for years, a more permanent form of soft tissue shortening called *contracture* can occur. In this case, the muscles may never again return to their normal resting length. Given enough time in this state, the cartilage and bones of the joint gradually succumb to the excess forces. They wear down and deform. This state of affairs, when found in the spine, is called *degenerative disc disease*. No amount of improvement of bony alignment or muscle balance will ever eliminate this degeneration and yet, as dire as this sounds, there may be some respite. If you minimize the misalignment and reduce the compression of the joints, you can diminish the effects of the existing condition and slow down, if not halt, the development of any further degeneration.

Our bodies' structural issues are keeping orthopedic surgeons busy, patching up the resulting knee and hip problems. I mention these operations because from my vantage point, too many hip and knee replacements are performed without the original offending misalignment ever being identified and rectified. This oversight contributes to the reinjury of more than 50% of surgical ACL (anterior cruciate ligament of the knee) repairs. Yes, the ACL has been properly sewn back together. And yes, the knee has been properly stretched and strengthened. But a crooked pelvis and its numerous complications make that knee an accident waiting to happen (again).

Here's an interesting case story that I like to share. Some years ago, a tai chi instructor visited my clinic because of unrelenting lower back and buttock pain that had been plaguing him for twenty-five years. During my assessment, I found his pelvis to be significantly posteriorly tilted. After I described what I saw in his body and why it was a problem, he told me that twenty-five years earlier, his sensei had instructed him to stand in a perpetual pelvic tilt (tailbone "tucked under") position. For all those years, he had abided by that advice and I could almost see the wheels turning in his head as he realized that by doing so, he'd been causing his own back pain. I confirmed that such advice might have helped someone with a pelvis that was already tilted too far forward. It would have brought that person's pelvis (and therefore their hips and spine) into a more neutral, more comfortable position. However, it was now apparent the instructor had not needed such advice. By way of his sensei's attempt to correct a problem that didn't exist, a very painful lower back was created.

Intervertebral Discs

I regularly see patients who've been told they have bulging or herniated discs. For some reason, there is a widespread notion that once you have a bulging or herniated disc, surgery is the only possible solution. It is not. Surgery is appropriate in many cases, but it is hardly ever the only solution. In fact, because traditional disc surgeries seldom address the underlying cause of the disc problem, they may not a real "solution" at all. Let's look a little more closely at the intervertebral disc (IVD) and see why this is true.

The primary function of the disc is to maintain adequate spacing between adjacent vertebrae. The spinal joints are positioned to enable them to function properly and to facilitate the entry and exit of nerves and blood vessels between the vertebrae. The discs also provide a certain amount of shock absorption for the spine.

An intervertebral disc is kind of like a jelly doughnut. There is a soft gelatinous center, surrounded by a tough, inelastic outer shell. The entire disc is anchored to the vertebrae, above and below, by strands of connective tissue. These attachments make it impossible for the disc to ever "go out of place". What can happen, however, is that the muscles, fascia and other soft tissues surrounding the spine can become so shortened, they force the disc to bulge out from between the vertebrae.

Imagine an Oreo cookie. The white center represents the disc and the two pieces of cookie represent the vertebrae. What happens to the soft center if you press the cookies together? It bulges outward, just as a disc bulges when the vertebrae are forced together.

How does a bulging disc differ from a herniated disc? A herniated disc occurs when the fibrous outer covering of the disc has actually ruptured. Your discs can withstand almost any amount of vertical compression without herniating. However, when a disc is so compressed there's no slack remaining in the outer covering, the addition of rotational force will cause tearing of the outer fibers. If enough of the outer fibers are broken, the soft inner core will be forced out through the tear. Imagine a jelly doughnut with a bite out of it. That's pretty much what a disc herniation looks like.

Both a bulging disc and a herniated one can be excruciatingly painful. Or they can be painless. It all depends on whether or not the protruding disc comes into contact with a pressure sensitive structure, like a nerve root. Nerve root compression commonly results in moderate to severe pain in one side of the lower back. The pain can continue down through the buttock, then to the back of the thigh and leg and sometimes, all the way down to the foot.

What can you do for a bulging or herniated disc? Since compression of the spine is almost always the underlying cause of these problems, anything that decompresses your spine will benefit your condition. There are numerous ways to accomplish this, ranging from sophisticated, computer-controlled traction tables to simple, active stretches. Keep in mind that your body is unlikely to release any muscle shortening until you have improved the underlying alignment problems. As long as you have not been saddled with an atypical complication, there will be at least one decompression technique that will prove to be appropriate for you. If you do so, I trust you'll approach your rehab process in a logical, orderly fashion in keeping with the Body Mechanic guidelines set out in this book.

The pain caused by a bulging or herniated disc might also be alleviated by trimming the disc and preventing it from compressing a nearby nerve. The surgery can provide wonderful relief but it's a Band-Aid solution. A temporary fix. So please, treat it accordingly. The surgery will buy you time to deal with the underlying issues that caused your disc problem. Since your newfound, pain-free post-surgical state will not last forever, take it as an opportunity to reorganize your body and guide it towards a more neutral posture. Perform relaxing movements, every day. Ease you muscles back, towards a state of equilibrium. Find your way to a mindset that offers you the probability of being pain-free.

One of the most common questions patients ask is whether or not their pain is due to a pinched nerve. Though nerves can be "pinched" (either compressed or entrapped), most pains that are assumed to be pressure on a nerve are most likely caused by a neuromuscular phenomenon called a *trigger point*. Here are the key differences between nerve compression, nerve entrapment and trigger points.

Nerve Compression

A nerve is said to be compressed when the pressure is caused by a bone or a soft tissue structure, such as a spinal disc. One of the most common examples of this phenomenon is when a nerve is compressed as it exits from between the bones of the spine. This type of compression can be due to a protruding disc, bony hypertrophy (extra bone deposited on the edge of a joint), or deviated positioning of one or more vertebrae.

Nerve Entrapment

A nerve is said to be entrapped when the pressure is caused by soft tissue, such as a muscle, that the nerve passes through. There are a few places in the body where this type of problem can occur, the most common being when the sciatic nerve is entrapped by the piriformis muscle (a muscle in the buttock). The sciatic nerve is the largest nerve in the body. Studies have proven that the sciatic nerve exits the pelvis beside the piriformis muscle in the majority of the people. It's generally agreed that somewhere between 10 and 20 percent of us possess a sciatic nerve that actually passes through the piriformis.

Anything that forces our piriformis muscle to be placed in a chronically tight position, either stretched or contracted, will almost certainly result in pressure being placed on the sciatic nerve. It's called 'compression' when the nerve travels beside the muscle and 'entrapment' when the nerve travels through the muscle. These are common origins of *sciatica*. This particular form of sciatica is called *piriformis syndrome*. The good news is that if you are able to teach your hips and pelvis to live in anything resembling a neutral position, the piriformis muscle won't have any reason to be either shortened or pulled taut. A relaxed piriformis muscle usually translates into "goodbye sciatica".

Trigger Points

Sometimes, people describe pain that doesn't seem to make sense. Why, when I apply pressure to a muscle in your upper back, would you feel pain in your head? What about that spot on your shoulder blade that makes you feel pain in your hand? People almost always assume these pains arise due to direct pressure on a nerve. However, these are just two of the most common examples of symptoms caused by *myofascial trigger points*.

A trigger point is a physiologically hypoactive area of tissue, usually muscle, that when stimulated becomes physiologically hyperactive. A trigger point can be stimulated (made painful) by compressing it or by muscle contraction. The primary characteristic that distinguishes a trigger point from any other sore, knotted area of muscle is called *referred sensation*. A sensation is 'referred' when it is felt somewhere other than where the trigger point is located. Each trigger point found in a person's body will refer sensation in a pattern or location that is unique. And yet, trigger points found in the same location in different people create surprisingly similar patterns of referred sensation. I know that sounds counterintuitive but that's how it is.

When we are talk about referred sensation we're usually talking about pain, but not always. An irritated trigger point can also cause feelings of numbness, tingling, cold, heat or weakness. Trigger points can result from a direct trauma to a muscle, or they can develop over time due to chronic overloading of tissues. Old injuries that have never been completely resolved, faulty movement patterns during work or exercise, and poor posture are all classic precursors of trigger point problems.

While it is not uncommon to have pain from either nerve compression or nerve entrapment, pain from trigger points is extremely common. In fact, trigger points are often responsible for the muscular shortening and alignment problems that result in nerve entrapment and nerve compression problems.

There are a number of trigger point treatment techniques. Arguably, the easiest and most effective technique is called *ischemic pressure*. Ischemic pressure is a sustained gentle pressure that is applied directly to the trigger point (with your finger, elbow, tennis ball, foam roll, etc.).

You press only hard enough to elicit moderate discomfort. A bonus feature of this technique is that it is something you can do yourself.

The trick to this technique is to apply enough pressure to stimulate the trigger point, but not so much that the body interprets the pressure as threatening (i.e. sharply painful). If you are doing it just right, the trigger point will start to relax out from under your pressure within 30 seconds. If you do not feel a lessening in the amount of discomfort within 30 seconds or so, then you are probably using too much pressure. Give it a few moments rest and try again with less pressure.

Some people find that preheating and post-treatment stretching enhance their ability to maintain the benefits obtained via the ischemic pressure technique. This is my favorite soft tissue treatment technique and it is a perfect complement to the Alignment First exercises.

This chapter has been all about how joint misalignment and muscle imbalance typically lead to painful compromises involving discs, nerves and trigger points. Until now, we have we have been developing a better understanding of lower back pain problems, but now it is time to take action. In the next chapter, we begin to explore the specific steps you can take in order to leave your pain where it belongs: in your past.

REMEMBER:

For some reason, there is a widespread notion that once you have a bulging or herniated disc, surgery is the only possible solution. It is not.

CHAPTER 6

What You Can Do About It

"Life isn't about finding yourself.
It's about creating yourself."
— GEORGE BERNARD SHAW

By this point, I trust you're seeing merit in becoming your own body mechanic. You've seen that many lower back pain problems can be solved and that most of them respond well to the do-it-yourself approach. Pain, especially lower back pain, is a contentious issue, but I've shared the concepts most experts can agree upon. I've debunked the myths about lower back pain, highlighted the obvious pain-causing issues and explained how they're expressed through the tissues of the body. Now it's time to start making good on the "you can do this" promise I made to you in Chapter One. It begins with this chapter identifying the things you can do to prepare your body to take advantage of the Alignment First Protocol.

A working knowledge of the issues relevant to the causes of lower back pain will help you understand the "why" of your problem. An acceptance of the importance of biomechanical alignment will help you determine "what to do" about your pain. That being said, a caution is in order regarding structural techniques that may have eased the discomfort of others. As interesting as hearsay can be, it is not therapeutic advice. Just because Active Release, IMS or Prolotherapy worked for a friend, that doesn't mean it will work for you. If you do try one of these therapies and don't experience the success your friend enjoyed, you won't know if your lack of success was because:

1. The brand of therapeutic intervention was inappropriate.
2. The brand of therapeutic intervention was appropriate but incomplete (i.e. requiring another, complimentary intervention to sufficiently address all your needs).
3. The brand of therapeutic intervention was appropriate but delivered unskillfully (i.e. recipe was right, but the cook screwed it up in the kitchen).
4. The brand of therapeutic intervention was appropriate, but the unique characteristics of your body resulted in a longer and more difficult journey from chronic pain to pain-free than your friend (i.e. on the right path, just not "there" yet).

Too many decisions about pain care are based on irrelevant information. Before choosing a technique to solve your lower back problem, it's important to understand the cause of your pain. If misalignment of your pelvis is the root cause of tension imbalances and spinal deviation, the chances of anything done to your lower back to resolve the cause of your problem, is pretty close to zero. Shockwave Therapy, ART and myofascial cupping, for example, may provide short-term relief. But because the source of your problem doesn't exist in your lower back, all you're doing is buying some time and delaying the inevitable. The underlying dysfunction will ultimately have its way with you.

The only logical way to proceed is to actually embark upon a biomechanical makeover. Training your body to become more efficient will naturally lead to less load on your body mechanically and neurologically.

Earlier in the book, I talked about your capacity to handle nervous system stimulation. I compared it to the memory on your smart phone and how many files it can hold. When it's close to full, it'll send you warning messages to avoid overloading your phone. That's what your body's doing when it sends you pain alarms. It's saying it's getting overloaded. So. What would you have to do in order to decrease the amount of neurological overload your lower back is trying to cope with? In addition, what would you have to do to also increase your body's capacity to cope with neurological input? Since these are the two most important questions you can ask yourself, the answers should shape how you proceed in caring for your chronic lower back pain problem.

No matter what stage you're at, in your journey towards lower back pain rehabilitation, this overview of the Alignment First Protocol will help you maximize the effectiveness of the process. Certain steps have to be taken on this path, and to maximize your success, these steps must be completed in the following sequence. The steps do overlap, but for clarity's sake we list them as separate and distinct. Think of this as your conceptual To-Do List:

1. Alignment—eliminate gross alignment problems (3 dimensionally)
2. Mobility—acquire normal ranges of motion in major weightbearing joints
3. Stability—improve your body's ability to resist force and maintain balance.
4. Motor Control—improve coordinated body movements.
5. Strength—increase your body's ability to apply force.
6. Endurance—increase how long you can sustain activity.

This list reflects the hierarchical importance of each element. As you have noticed by now, I talk a fair bit about how improved alignment tends to improve other functions in your body. That's why alignment is the first and most important measure of both your current situation and of your progress.

Once the major alignment issues are cleared off the table, you'll shift your emphasis to mobility. It's amazing how muscle imbalances, that interfere with adequate mobility, can wreak havoc on the functional abilities and comfort of your body. Mobility is about training your body, maybe for the first time ever, to move your major weightbearing joints through a full range of motion that's considered normal and healthy.

Once you begin seeing mobility improvements, it'll be time to pay attention to your stability and to the quality of your movements. We're not prepping you for the Olympics, but you do need to perform certain fundamental movement patterns in a safe, controlled manner.

One of the great yardsticks for this purpose is the deep squat. Can you keep your feet parallel when you squat? Can you keep your heels on the ground and get your hips below your knees? When you do squat, can you prevent your knees from coming together? Are you able to keep your spine in a somewhat neutral position? Most people are able to do all of the above, but only when they hold onto something to increase their stability. If that's also the case for you, know that you're in the majority. With practice, you'll be able to do this exercise properly, but don't let your early efforts discourage you. In the beginning, most people can't do a squat well, even when hanging on for support. This highlights the fact that in order to develop significant motor control, you need to establish stability and a stable base of support, along with the ability to transfer that stability further up in your body.

Strength and endurance, to the extent that they are required for our purposes, are a natural and desirable consequence of the protocol exercises.

You don't need to be an expert to discern what your imbalances are. You can determine if your asymmetry is on the left or right side of your body. You can also tell if alignment is your problem. To a reasonable degree, you can also evaluate your own mobility, movement quality, strength and endurance abilities. If the essence of rehabilitation is to figure out what your body is doing poorly and then train it to do those things better, then Alignment First is an excellent program to follow. Over time, the protocol will guide you towards the systematic elimination of your imbalances.

And whether you have aspirations beyond eliminating your chronic lower back pain or not, the protocol benefits just about everyone. It doesn't matter whether you are a waitress or a weightlifter, an orchestra or a train conductor, 99 years old or 19, the principles are the same. Get straighter, then get more mobile. Move better and then get stronger. The step-by-step progression of this process is the same for everyone.

Here are some rehab treatments that I teach patients, to help them maximize their results with the Alignment First exercises:

Ice or heat?

When people experience pain, just about everyone asks, "should I use ice or heat?" Traditionally, when there were signs of inflammation, such as heat, redness and/or swelling, we used the classic I.C.E. prescription. I.C.E. stands for *Ice*, *Compression* and *Elevation*. Compression (wrapping) and elevation (getting the swollen body part literally higher than the heart) are considered useful strategies for reducing fluid congestion and lessening the related discomfort. The use of ice, however, is not enjoying the respect it once had.

Ice

The theory was that ice would cause a contraction of the small muscles within the blood vessels in the swollen area, thereby reducing swelling and pain. But because ice can retard fluid flow in the tissues, people wanting faster swelling reduction are opting for the more efficient on-again, off-again, pumping action of repeated muscle contractions. This practice has led to fewer professionals instructing people to use ice to control pain and swelling of injured or chronically irritated tissues.

Ice does have a pain reducing effect, which is still a valuable characteristic. Some people still suggest alternating heat and cold, as a way to try to decrease swelling without creating *stasis* (reduction or stoppage of fluid flow) in the tissues. Though the science seems to support this practice, hardcore "no ice" proponents insist that the use of ice should go the way of the dinosaur.

Originally, the prescription was actually R.I.C.E. (Rest, Ice, Compression, Elevation). Rest has since been placed upon the sidelines as well. Certainly, you need to respect your pain. That message will never change. However, even if you don't feel that you can get out of bed, you may still be able to do some gentle movements. Pelvic Tilts or Single Leg Bent Knee Raises may help decrease tissue congestion and related pain. Current research clearly suggests that absolute bedrest and immobility are rarely the best option. As a long-time believer in the benefits of pain-free movement, whether standing, sitting or lying down, I am pleased to see that scientific evidence continues to support that idea.

The modern and more appropriate prescription may now be M.I.C.E (Movement, Heat/Ice, Compression, Elevation). I have used this strategy with much success, though I have not abandoned the icepack quite yet. Should you choose to use ice, be conservative. When alternating between ice and heat, I encourage my patients to use ice for fifteen minutes, followed by five minutes of heat. But please note: this is not a universal prescription. When using ice, more isn't necessarily better. And in the presence of acute inflammation, five minutes of heat will almost certainly be too long.

No matter how you choose to proceed, the important thing is to minimize swelling, whenever it is possible. There is an abundance of research that demonstrates how joint inflammation can interfere with efficient motor control in the muscles that cross the joint in question. So, what's "the bottom line"? Use gentle movement of the area, if you are able to, and use my preceding ramblings to help guide your own experimentation. Find out what works for you, because that is ultimately your best course of action. You know how your body feels better than anyone else. So be like a chef in the kitchen and "season to taste". Your taste.

Heat

When there is no obvious evidence of inflammation, heat can increase blood flow and neuromuscular relaxation in the painful area. A hot bath, a hot water bottle, or an electric heating pad can be effective in warming and relaxing the tissues. Heating these tissues, prior to stretching, can maximize your results. Indeed, I've seen quite a few people receive tremendous value from doing their stretching in a hot tub.

However, if your discomfort increases after heating up your lower back, take it as a sign that you're on the wrong track. Experiment with yourself. Discontinue the heat and pay attention to how your body responds. If that change of direction doesn't seem to help, you may need to change tactics and get "old school". By that I mean, pull out the ice pack and give it a try. Be inquisitive and mindful of how your body reacts. Your ability to read and react to the messages your body sends, will help you become more comfortable with this process.

Compression

When your lower back is the painful, inflamed area, it is awkward to wrap or compress your waist to limit swelling. At first glance, there seem to be quite a selection of bandages, back braces and belts to support and compress the lower back. Usually, however, when people do use a belt or back brace, they're doing it for added stability, not for limiting inflammation. Still and all, you could wrap your ice pack or heating pad in an elastic bandage and use that to hold it in place and thereby, enhance the compression element of your efforts.

As a bit of an aside, a compression strategy called "flossing" or "voodoo flossing" is gaining traction in the sports performance community. Kelly Starrett (an expert on human movement and mobility) is a proponent of this technique, and he, and others as well, have YouTube videos demonstrating this way of applying therapeutic compression. Although I have not seen it used much to minimize inflammation in the lower back, it's a good way to limit inflammation and restore mobility to peripheral joints such as the hip, knee and ankle. And usually, anything that improves the mobility of these joints contributes to the relief of chronic lower back pain.

Elevation

When adding the elevation element to the equation, you are raising the swollen body part above the heart. This will improve circulation from the swollen area back to the heart and accelerate the draining of the inflammation, from the injured and irritated area. Like the issue of compression, elevation is rarely used as a tactic to minimize swelling in the lower back. However, swelling in peripheral joints such as ankles or knees can be decreased by simply getting on your back and putting your legs up a wall. As mentioned in the preceding section, the better these joints perform, the better it is for your lower back.

Mobilization

When I got out of college in 1989, stretching was the only way to self-mobilize. Then, a few years later, I was introduced to the idea of using of a pool noodle to improve positioning during floor exercise. A year or two after that, I used a foam roll as a form of self-massage for the first time. Today, objects of all shapes, sizes and materials are being used to mobilize soft tissues and joints.

I teach all my patients how to use floor exercises for self-care. As for which tools and props are best for self-care, I take my lead from renowned physiotherapists Kelly Starrett and Brian Mulligan. I'm also beginning to like what Donnie Thompson, a strength and mobility expert, is up to.

Dr. Kelly Starrett, a physical therapist in San Francisco, is regarded as one of the world's foremost experts on human movement and mobility. He uses all kinds of bands and balls for self-mobilization and he offers excellent, how-to instructions and videos on his website at thereadystate.com. Many of these videos are also available on YouTube.

Brian Mulligan is a physiotherapist from New Zealand. He has been teaching his particular brand of mobilization and self-mobilization since the 1970s. Brian's work involves using an inelastic strap to pull joints out of positions of strain, and into positions of ease. It's easy to see Brian's influence in the work of younger experts, such as Kelly Starrett. There are also a number of YouTube videos that demonstrate Brian's techniques.

Body Tempering is the latest technique for self-mobilization. It was developed by Donnie Thompson, the first man to ever lift a combined, three thousand pounds in the three powerlifts (deadlift, squat and bench press) in a competition. He reached the peak of his illustrious career as a powerlifter in his late 40s. As one of the greatest strength athletes of all time, he attributes much of his longevity and his relatively injury-free journey to his discovery of what he calls Body Tempering.

Essentially, this is to use one or more heavy steel rods to massage the body, like a foam roll does. The difference is in the placement of the two tools. With a foam roll, we are typically moving our body on top of the roll. When body tempering, the steel rod is placed and moved, on top of our body. Donnie's original steel rod weighed 135 pounds. Since then he has experimented with many different sizes and weights of rods. Check out Donnie's website at www.bodytempering.com to learn more. He also has a number of videos on YouTube.

If you decide to experiment with Donnie's techniques, please proceed with due care and attention. If you are new to self-mobilization, I strongly suggest that you fully explore the Mulligan and Starrett strategies before looking at what Donnie Thompson is up to. I think that Donnie's strategies are excellent. In fact, I use body tempering myself. But without professional supervision, this is not where you should begin.

1. Foam Roll

Think of the foam roll as being a rolling pin and your body as the dough. You're going to lie down, on top of the roll, and move yourself over it, giving yourself a form of self-massage. This technique helps to increase local circulation. It can locate trigger points in the soft tissues and help decrease excessive muscle tone. It is a great way to begin your self-treatment session, because a fundamental concept of therapy is to begin your treatment broadly and then, narrow it down gradually, becoming more specific as you go. The foam roll helps you do this.

Another use for the foam roll is as a fulcrum. You can lie on it to create a pivot point that lets you bend your body in a way that you might not otherwise be able to do. For example, if your spine is chronically flexed, your upper back and ribcage are probably quite stiff. With your knees bent, lie on your back on the floor, on top of the roll. Place the roll at the apex of the curve in your spine. Breathe slowly and deeply and do your best to just let gravity do its thing. This mobilization technique can be surprisingly powerful, as it often reveals a shortness in the soft tissues of the abdomen and shoulder girdles.

2. Body Tempering

As I mentioned earlier, the Body Tempering technique, invented by Donnie Thompson, is similar to using a foam roll, but also different. The similarities are in how they both help to compress and create movement between different layers of tissues. Deep connective tissues, muscles and superficial fascia are smashed and moved independently.

As you can imagine, a heavy steel rod can compress the tissues and move fluids, within the body, to a degree not attainable with a foam roll. The procedure provides an impressive degree of relaxation of the treated muscles that I've never seen or experienced with foam rolls. But because Body Tempering is in its infancy, we're proceeding with care. It is clear that this is one way to deliver a very broad form of ischemic pressure. But the details of how the body responds neuro-physiologically, to the forceful movement of fluid out of the tissues, has yet to be defined. My experiments with Body Tempering, on my own body and on patients, have been largely successful, so I'm looking forward to gathering more experience and expertise.

3. Exercise Band

The exercise band I refer to is essentially a modern, heavy duty descendent of a classic rubber band. You can purchase these bands at any exercise equipment store. They are well known and commonly used in the athletic training world. And they're becoming a popular tool in the more traditional rehab circles. The bands can be particularly useful when you are trying to teach joints, such as shoulders or hips, to assume a more neutral position. You can see the bands at work in a number of online Kelly Starrett videos that demonstrate how to effectively use this strategy.

4. Mulligan Strap

The type of inelastic strap that Brian Mulligan uses for his particular brand of self-mobilization is a specialty item that can be purchased through medical equipment supply stores. Mulligan Mobilization is widely known within the professional rehabilitation community, but largely unknown otherwise. There are videos demonstrating these techniques on YouTube and Brian's book titled *Manual Therapy: NAGS, SNAGS MWMS, etc.* is a terrific resource, if you are interested in learning more about this particular approach.

5. Therapy Ball

The humble tennis ball was the original therapy ball but today, it's just one of many variations available. I have a handful of therapy balls at my office. No matter their size or their density, they're all great self-treatment tools, partly because their effective use can be so easily taught. You can use them when seated. Put the ball between your foot and the floor. Or put it between the chair and your glute or hamstrings. Stand up and you can put the ball between your chest or shoulder and the wall. Or do what I encourage most of my patients to do: lie down on the ball and move over it.

No matter what position you use, you're trying to find those tight and uncomfortable soft tissues that are not only responsible for restricted circulation and joint mobility, they're also often sources of pain. Once you have found the offending soft tissues, try to place the ball in the most acutely sensitive location and adjust your pressure so that it yields an amount of discomfort that you are able to relax into. If the discomfort is not excessive, you should feel a lessening of the tenderness within thirty seconds. If it hasn't lessened within that time, I suggest that you try a different location. When you are applying the right amount of pressure, in an appropriate location, it is not unusual for the discomfort to begin lessening within ten seconds or less.

If the tissues are more tight and hard than acutely sensitive, there is another technique you can use that can work wonders. What you do is anchor those tissues to your underlying skeleton with the ball. Then, when you move the adjacent joint, you're producing a do-it-yourself form of Active Release Technique. This is an excellent way to resolve stubborn mobility restrictions. I've found it particularly effective when trying to mobilize the shoulder, hip and ankle. As mentioned previously, by improving their mobilization, you're contributing to the relief of your chronic lower back pain problem.

A third type of ball work is to lie on your stomach and use a soft ball to minimize muscle guarding in the abdominal area. For this purpose, a tennis ball or lacrosse ball is usually too small. I've experimented with balls of all sizes and found that a volleyball with a little air taken out of it or a similarly-sized, department-store kid's ball works best.

This ball therapy seems to accomplish several things simultaneously. It tends to take your lumbar spine out of hyperextension by mechanically moving it into a more neutral position. It also delivers some ischemic pressure to the abdominal muscles, which may very well be housing a trigger point or two. And since some experts believe abdominal trigger points contribute to lower back pain problems, this might be an added bonus.

I mention that when it comes to releasing trigger points, I'm not stuck on treating them with a sharp elbow, thumb or syringe. I know that broad, gentle pressure can work quite well, if location and breathing are appropriate. And I want to add that getting on top of an underinflated soccer ball, allows you the opportunity to try a technique that has been popularized by body whisperer and pain eraser, Jill Miller, PT. She is a proponent of alternately contracting and relaxing the tight muscles in your core. You take a large breath and push your abdominal muscles into the ball for a couple seconds, then exhale and relax into the ball as much as possible. And then repeat. This might also be an appropriate time to experiment with the diaphragmatic breathing techniques discussed further on, in this chapter. Working on your breathing technique only takes a couple of minutes of your time and since it often yields good results, it's worth a try.

Movement Re-education

The first book I read after graduating from massage therapy college was Thomas Hanna's *Somatics: Reawakening the Mind's Control of Movement, Flexibility, and Health* (1988 Da Capo Press). In my opinion, this is still one of the best books about physical self-care. Mr. Hanna presents an easy to understand explanation for common dysfunctional postural patterns. He grounds it with some fascinating case histories and then brings it all together with a series of floor exercise routines, designed to optimize both posture and physical function. He coined the term "sensory-motor amnesia" to describe how we sometimes literally forget how to coordinate healthy motor function, in response to the sensory signals we receive from our environment. His "somatic" exercises were designed to restore that lost sensory awareness and motor control. I highly recommend his book to anyone who is interested in this subject. In many ways, it's a perfect complement to what we're talking about here, in my book.

Another approach to neuromuscular re-education is Dynamic Neuromuscular Stabilization, which was developed by Dr. Pavel Kolar, PT. As a physiotherapist by training and with a doctorate in pediatrics, it's no surprise his approach is based on the idea that children develop motor skills in a predictable sequence. By strategically stimulating these fundamental developmental programs in the body, we can improve function.

As an approach, DNS has become very popular and is now being used by many of the most respected practitioners in the rehab world. Although there are no books yet available on do-it-yourself DNS exercises, I expect there soon will be. In the meantime, there are healthcare practitioners trained in DNS techniques.

While the exercise band is well used for joint mobilization and repositioning, it's also very useful for retraining motor control. For example, if you're doing a squat and have difficulty keeping one of your knees from moving toward the other, you can use the band to improve this biomechanical fault. Anchor the band to something stationary, such as a heavy piece of furniture or a door handle. Place the other end of the band around the outside of the knee, on the side you wish to retrain. Move your body far enough away from the anchored end of the band, so that there is considerable tension in the band. Now, when you squat down, the band will be pulling your knee inward, which is an exaggeration of the dysfunctional movement pattern. You will have to fight that tension by pulling outward with your hip muscles, in order to produce a decent movement pattern. Practice of this exercise will gradually improve your motor control in that previously unstable hip/knee. It will also enhance your skill in the basic squat movement pattern. And by the way, if both of your knees are determined to turn toward each other, the same procedure can used on each. (But separately, of course.)

Balance

I am against advocating specific balance training too early in the rehab process. But once alignment and mobility are being managed, there is a place for this kind of intervention. And there are ample tools that can be used for this purpose.

A simple way to begin is to practice your deep squat. It's great for balance, whether it's a static pose or an active movement. But remember what I said about squats earlier: the vast majority of people are initially unable to assume a deep squat position with anything resembling a full range of motion. It's a fact: most people are unable to demonstrate healthy positional relationships between their major weightbearing joints. But don't let that make you spurn the squat. When people are allowed to hang onto a heavy piece of furniture or a door frame for added stability, the majority are able to assume a reasonable facsimile of the desired positioning. And better yet, almost all get better with practice.

Another simple and "easy" way to include balance training within your program is to begin standing on one leg. Later, you can practice standing on one leg with your eyes closed. But do the eyes-closed version within a doorframe, or beside a counter, so you can grab onto something if you do lose your balance. (It happens!) There are a number of other ways you can safely increase the training demands from there. But please, do ignore the videos on YouTube that show people doing barbell squats on exercise balls. The risks associated with these practices are, I think, pretty obvious.

Diaphragmatic Breathing

For thousands of years, various forms of breathing practice have been taught through yoga and martial arts systems. I believe that's because most of us need to learn how to breathe in a healthier way. We tend to inhale by using the muscles of our ribcage, chest and neck. But that's not the primary job of those muscles. Yes, they're designed to assist in the mechanics of breathing, but they are not supposed to be doing all the heavy lifting. By using those muscles to drive respiration, we're detracting from their ability to perform their primary jobs properly.

The big engine of breathing should be your diaphragm and for some very some good reasons, too. Diaphragmatic breathing is a great tool for interrupting the pain-tension cycle and for calming the nervous system. Proper breathing techniques contribute to mobilization by helping normalize spine and ribcage alignment and mobility. Plus, proper breathing may be considered a form of stability training due to how it can improve activation of deep core muscles.

A common breathing practice recommendation is to breathe in and out through your nose, 5 to 7 times per minute. By purposefully slowing down your breathing, you're stimulating the parasympathetic nervous system (our rest and recovery neurology) as opposed to the sympathetic nervous system (our fight or flight neurology). Some people believe we should strive to function this way at all times and others suggest that it is something to be done only in times of pain and or stress.

One system of breathing that probably originated in India and is widely taught in yoga classes around the world, is to breathe in through your nose and exhale through your mouth. Hold the tip of your tongue on the roof of your mouth just behind your teeth. Begin by inhaling for four seconds. Hold your breath for seven seconds. Then exhale for eight seconds. Repeat these three steps four times.

Dr. Andrew Weil, the world-renowned health guru, is a vocal proponent of this technique which he calls "4-7-8 breathing". He has numerous videos online explaining it in greater detail. He suggests that people practice this breathing technique daily, gradually building up to doing two separate sessions of the four breath cycles, to equal the maximum recommended dose of eight sets of this exercise per day. Experiment with it and see what you think. Know that if you are an extremely shallow breather, any new breathing strategy will typically be challenging. It may feel scary when you hold your lungs without air in them for even a second or two. Give it time, however, and that panicky feeling will dissipate. Meanwhile, you'll be reducing the load on your nervous system, just by changing how you breathe.

The breathing exercises that Thomas Hanna teaches in his book *Somatics,* are radically different from most others. His approach involves holding your breath and then shifting that held air, first up and down in your torso and then diagonally. I think of it as push-ups for your diaphragm. Hanna's procedure is an effective re-education strategy, both in terms of enabling more relaxed breathing and also in increasing mobility of the torso.

Once you master diaphragmatic breathing, you will have taken an enormous step towards exerting conscious control over your nervous system. Given the overarching importance of the nervous system and the key role that oxygen plays in physiology, diaphragmatic breathing may actually be the fastest, most efficient way to improve whole body health. If you insert one of the preceding breathing exercises into your daily schedule, morning and night, I'm betting you'll be glad you did.

This has been a wide-ranging chapter because of the many different ways you can prepare your body to maximize the benefits of the Alignment First Protocol. I urge you to begin working on your breathing and start practicing your deep squat as you move on to the next chapter. It provides a practical level of advice to help you implement the protocol successfully.

REMEMBER:

Get straighter, then get more mobile. Move better and then get stronger.

Diaphragmatic breathing may actually be the fastest, most efficient way to improve whole body health.

CHAPTER 7

How You Can Do It

*"People often say that motivation doesn't last. Well, neither
does bathing—that's why we recommend it daily."*
— Zig Ziglar

The following guidelines evolved while I was developing the Alignment First Protocol. If you treat them as touchstones, they'll help you perform the protocol's step-by-step exercises that correct the common biomechanical issues that lead to lower back pain.

You will notice that most of the exercises used in the protocol are generally considered to be stretches, even though there is often very little stretching involved. Paired muscles and muscle groups, such as the quadriceps and hamstrings, pull on opposite sides of the same bony structures, in a perpetual tug-of-war relationship. For example, if your pelvis is rotated too far forward, you will find your hamstrings pulled taut and your quadriceps/hip flexors shortened. Prior to reading this book, you might have wanted to stretch those tight-feeling hamstrings. But now, you know that stretching almost never creates slack and/or lasting comfort in the hamstrings. Relief will not happen when those muscles are already pulled taut.

However, if you stretch the quadriceps/hip flexors, one or both of the following things will happen. Ideally, the quadriceps/hip flexors will relax and lengthen somewhat. And even if nothing else happens, that lengthening of these muscles will lessen the tension and result in greater mobility in that hip. Granted, this will not guarantee a more neutral pelvic position. (But wait, there's more!) If the hamstrings have not been excessively weakened by chronic tautness, the tug-of-war between the two muscle groups should rotate the pelvis back into a more neutral position. That repositioning of the pelvis is a major improvement. Should there also be lengthening of the shortened quadriceps and hip flexor muscles, then so much the better.

And now, since the protocol is so much about stretching, here's the long and the short of it.

Stretching

My go-to source on stretching is called *The Stark Reality of Stretching*. Written by Dr. Steven Stark, this book is overflowing with scientific research references that support his assertion that gentle, sustained stretching is the most efficient method for lengthening shortened muscles. If your interest in stretching exceeds what I'm about to share on the subject, Dr. Stark's book has my strongest recommendation. I've never met anyone who knows more about stretching or, for that matter, more about foot and ankle function, either.

What is a stretch?

College students in first-year anatomy and physiology classes might tell you that a stretch in a muscle occurs when the overlapping protein fibers of the muscle cells slide past each other in the direction that elongates the muscle.

This simple definition is easy to understand but unfortunately, it doesn't apply to all stretches. Many do not result in an elongation of the target muscle/muscle group at all. Other stretches, due to errors of technique and/or exercise choice, can actually harm muscle and/or joint structures. Stretching too aggressively can work against maintaining muscle length gains. That's because, if every time you stretch you also trigger the stretch reflex, your body tightens in self defense. This reflex makes it difficult for you to effect lasting range of motion improvements. Just to be clear, the stretch reflex is a natural contraction of the muscle in response to a sudden, or strong, pull on the muscle.

Some stretches may lengthen the muscle, but only temporarily. This reaction is usually less about anything specific regarding the stretch; it's more about your body not feeling safe enough to surrender the muscular bracing it has been maintaining. It's holding back for your own good.

Why stretch?

The short answer is, use it or lose it. As you get older, it becomes ever more important for you to have a daily movement regimen. It's the best way to maintain good structural alignment and a healthy range of motion in your joints. Your major weightbearing joints (ankles, knees, hips and spine) were meant to last a lifetime. If you take care of them, they will take care of you. A daily stretching routine, that you can live with for the longer haul, will keep you in the game.

I know how boring the prospect of a daily stretching routine can sound. But given that the alternative is chronic pain that you could have avoided, I'd opt to give it a serious try. I can almost guarantee you will feel better. And given the prevalence of adaptive shortening, you might even sleep better, too.

Adaptive shortening? It's a natural process of muscle tightening that we're all subject to. It continues 24/7 and we would be completely unaware of it, if we were physically active enough to regularly move all of our joints through a full range of motion. But most of us are not that active on a consistent basis.

That's why everyone needs a variety of ongoing movements to stay physically healthy. If your normal daily activities don't provide enough physical mobility opportunities, then you need to set aside some time and develop a movement practice that works for you. It's simply a matter of body maintenance. Stretch first to organize your body into a healthier posture. Stretch second to turn that posture into healthier mobility. And finally, stretch to maintain the benefits you're getting from your improved posture and mobility.

One last note: here's an example of adaptive shortening. It occurs when your arm is in a sling due to a forearm fracture. If you neglect to regularly straighten your elbow as it heals, it will become very difficult to straighten. That's because, over time, the muscles that flex your elbow have gradually shortened to reflect how your body has recently been used. Or in this case, not used.

Which muscles should I stretch?

I am a big advocate of mobility programs that deliver lasting benefits. For that to happen, the process must bring about improvements in alignment before anything else. I am wholeheartedly committed to this alignment first stance because there are basic patterns of alignment that we can use as reference points.

We humans may be as unique as snowflakes on the outside. But on the inside, our physiologies are remarkably similar, especially as they relate to the issues surrounding the more common causes of lower back pain. These similarities enable us to guide our dysfunctional bodies toward a common baseline of alignment and function. It works well for almost all of us but yes, I am sorry to say, if your physiology falls on the extreme ends of the bell curve, relative to the rest of us, you will not find the answers to your problems in this book. Or any other, I expect.

Earlier in my career, I wanted to test the joint range of motion of every new patient. I felt it was important to figure out each patient's primary movement restriction. As time passed, however, I found that when people practice the Alignment First Protocol, their basic alignment almost always changes, as do their mobility numbers. I've also found that by customizing the protocol less and by simply letting the process work its magic, the same exercises, in case after case, seem to be the most impactful. Like so many other processes, it indeed appears that the whole of the protocol is greater than just the sum of its parts.

Functional assessments, performed after the changes take place, are almost always more revealing and more meaningful than the mobility measurements taken beforehand. This observation has reinforced my belief in the importance of normalizing the alignment of the skeleton. It is the first and most important step in rehabbing any chronic pain problem.

So now, when people ask, "what should I stretch first?", my response is more of an explanation than a simple answer. Historically, the rule was: you stretch the muscle responsible for the biggest dysfunction, whether that was alignment, mobility or discomfort. Nowadays, my recommendation is to get good at the Alignment First Protocol because it will change your perspective on what your biggest dysfunction is. I can almost guarantee that it will be different from what you perceived your dysfunction to be, before you began your exercises. This self-customizing characteristic of the Alignment First Protocol will help you point yourself in the right direction.

How long should I hold the stretch?

The most asked question about stretching is, "How long should I hold the stretch?". This has led to much debate amongst healthcare and athletic training experts. This how-long-to-stretch issue has also led to a great deal of research about muscle function, with the consensus being: there is no single optimal timeframe for holding a stretch. Here's why:

The most efficient way to stretch begins by starting with no tension in the target muscle. Then, you slowly move into a position where you can sense some stretch tension in the targeted muscle. You hold that position until you feel that initial tension disappearing. To gain more length, you then repeat this process. Keep it gentle. If you stretch the target muscle aggressively, you will set off the stretch reflex (a contraction of the muscle in response to either a sudden or strong pull on it). When that happens, the muscle can't lengthen until the reflex contraction relaxes and the muscle is allowed to return to its original resting length.

The above procedure is scientifically proven to be the most efficient and effective method of stretching. But as simple as it sounds, most people are not accustomed to paying such close attention to their body sensations. It's been my experience that many people just don't have the patience and dedication necessary to use this method successfully.

For that reason, I almost always ask my patients and protocol participants to hold their stretches for one minute. When people adhere to this approach, they are unlikely to stretch so aggressively that they overstretch or injure themselves. And though there is no research to support the one-minute hold approach, most people seem ready, willing and able to apply the method to their stretching efforts. More importantly, it seems to work for them and contribute to their success.

Should you prefer to get the absolute maximum benefit out of each stretching moment, then I encourage you to utilize the least sensation/

first awareness approach and put away your stopwatch. To learn even more about the science of stretching, get a copy of *The Stark Reality of Stretching* by Dr. Steven Stark.

Now let's add to your understanding of the fundamentals of stretching by reviewing the most common stretching mistakes:

1. Not Warming Up Prior to Stretching

You already know you should engage in some kind of warm up activity prior to exercising. For stretching and mobilization routines, a warm up will increase blood flow and literally warm the soft tissues of the body. That will improve the ability of your muscles to relax and elongate. A brisk walk, some jumping jacks or a hot bath are just some of the ways to prepare your muscles in order to maximize the benefits of your stretching and mobilization practice. If you experiment with a few warm up activities, you'll find a method that works for you.

2. Stretching "Too Hard"

Using too much force, while attempting to stretch a muscle, usually triggers the stretch reflex, a neuromuscular automatic response that functions as a self defense mechanism. When sensors in the tendon feel an excessively abrupt or strong pull, the muscle is triggered to shorten. It's trying to protect itself against injury and that's good. But the drawback, to this contraction, is how it prevents the kind of relaxation and elongation you need in the muscle, to facilitate any kind of sustainable lengthening. Instead, all you get is the rubber band effect: a temporary stretching and a subsequent shortening. It's as if you expanded a rubber band and then let it shrink back, again.

Research and experience have taught us that the static stretch-and-hold procedure is a safe and effective method of stretching. However, I continue to see people using *ballistic stretches*. A stretch is called ballistic when you bounce in and out of the stretch position. Because ballistic stretches trigger the stretch reflex, they are not efficient for increasing tissue length.

The strong, abrupt pulling of the muscles and tendons, associated with ballistic stretching, can lead to muscle strains and in extreme cases, even tendon and joint injuries. Some folks believe that if the amount of force is reduced so that the "stretch" is no longer likely to injure, then it may no longer be dangerous. If pursued within rational limits, such movements can be used as a warm up strategy. When used accordingly, they're often called *dynamic stretches*, but don't be misled by that name. These movements are not stretches.

Have you heard the term *active stretching*? It applies to the kind of stretching you do on your own. *Passive stretching* is when you have someone else stretch you. *Active-assisted stretching* is when you stretch as far as you can and then someone else provides *overpressure* to move you further than you could ever move under your own power. In most cases, the use of overpressure is not a good idea. Should you insist on indulging, I urge you to ensure the person helping you stretch is an expert in this field, or you will regret not doing so.

Even if you are working with a stretching expert, be extremely careful and maintain constant communication during the process. No matter how much of an expert he/she may be, they can never feel what is happening inside your body. Only you can do that. And whatever you do, don't let anyone talk you into a "no pain, no gain" approach to stretching.

If you are the kind of person who tends toward the "no pain, no gain" approach to the challenges in your life, please set that attitude aside while you deal with your lower back. Pushing through that pain will only lead to more suffering. If, at any time, an exercise causes you to feel acute pain, please stop immediately. And don't do anything that increases your pain, even if you've been told by an expert that it's okay; that what you're trying to do is correct. If you encounter pain, try easing up on the amount of pressure you're using. If that doesn't decrease your discomfort, then move on to the next exercise. You can always try again tomorrow. After all, postural reorganization is a marathon not a sprint. And remember: almost all of the research says that low force, long duration, static stretching yields the best results.

3. Not Focusing Enough Attention on the Muscle You Are Trying to Stretch

The real secret to effective stretching is to be completely focused on the sensation in the target muscle while you're attempting to stretch it. It helps to understand what's supposed to happen within the muscle in order for it to actually lengthen (and not just stretch and then snap back like a rubber band). When you're focused enough on the tension in the muscle while you're performing the stretch, you'll be able to sense how much tension is necessary to allow the muscle to relax and lengthen. And as you practice this approach to stretching, you will find that your neuromuscular system is gradually learning how to allow your muscles to relax and stretch more quickly and easily, as time goes by.

4. Poor Positioning

There are two key issues concerning poor positioning for a stretch. The first is when you are positioned in such a way that you are placing abnormal stress on a joint. The most common example of this is the classic *hurdler's stretch*. It's supposed to be a hamstring stretch. But here's what happens. While you're focused on stretching the hamstrings on one side of your body, you may be placing dangerous stress on the opposite knee. Shin Box is another stretch that can be useful, but extra caution is required to ensure it is practiced safely. For the best and safest results, always stretch in a pain-free range of motion.

The second positioning issue, and ironically the one most commonly overlooked, has to do with putting yourself in a position that literally prevents the target muscle from ever being able to relax and elongate. For this reason, almost all standing stretches for the muscles of the lower body are suspect. When you perform a standing hamstring stretch, for example, how can your hamstrings relax and elongate when they are being used at the same time, to hold you up against the pull of gravity? Even the standing quadriceps stretch is not a particularly efficient stretch. True, the thigh you are stretching is not bearing any weight. But the problem is with the quadriceps on the other side of your body. They're now supporting all of your weight so they're telling on you: they're sending out a neurological SOS to the muscles you are trying to stretch. It's counterproductive. A better idea is to switch to one of the non-weightbearing versions of this stretch.

5. Stretching the "Wrong" Muscle(s)

Upon feeling any kind of muscle tightness, it's normal to assume that the muscle needs to be stretched. That assumption can be a mistake because it's just as common for a muscle to feel tight because it is pulled taut, as opposed to actually being shortened. And obviously, if the muscle in question is tight because it is being held in a stretched position, stretching it further won't help. In such a scenario, the actual culprit is the shortened muscle(s) that is pulling the tight-feeling muscle into its lengthened position. This shortened muscle is the one that needs to be stretched, if any lasting muscle balance and comfort is to be achieved.

Two common examples of this phenomenon include the hamstrings and chest muscles. I've already mentioned how often people want to stretch their hamstrings when actually, they should be stretching their shortened quadriceps. A similar imbalance occurs in your chest muscles and the muscles between your shoulder blades. It is very common for chronically short chest and upper abdominal muscles to overpower and weaken the muscles between your shoulder blades.

This imbalance typically causes the shoulders to be pulled forward and down, resulting in complaints of chronic shoulder, upper back and neck discomfort. In such cases, stretching the upper back, neck and rotator cuff muscles will not work. Relief will only come when the muscles of the chest and anterior shoulders have been lengthened, thus allowing the upper body to return to a more neutral, more comfortable posture.

I add that a lot of muscle shortening is created, intentionally by the body, as a means of stabilizing a weak and/or unstable segment of the body. For example, if you're about to ask your inner thigh muscles to stretch out while your body is purposely tightening them to stabilize your pelvis and/or thighs, you're going to have a struggle that's unavoidable.

It is worth noting that though many people refer to their exercises as "my stretches", the First Alignment program of exercises is designed to reorganize the body positionally. Many of them even have the word "stretch" in their name, but their value to us, in this approach, is how they help us to position the body in a more balanced, neutral position. It is this improved position which helps the body adapt to and cope with the stresses of life.

6. Frequency

I ask my patients to practice their corrective exercises once a day, to begin with. Sometimes the body is not eager to welcome the postural re-organization that these exercises promote. In these instances, it almost seems as though the body is "afraid" to change. A physical example of fear-of-the-unknown.

To minimize this issue, I've found it prudent to begin with one corrective exercise session a day. If your body hasn't complained about the demands of your new exercise regimen after a week or two, you can begin doing the exercises twice daily. But this is an option that is entirely up to you. I want you to know that many people get all the benefits they need from practicing their exercises once a day. But I do add that it isn't hard to imagine that doing them twice a day could accelerate progress.

Be cognizant of the fact that there seems to be a steadily diminishing benefit, in regard to adding more sessions. And keep in mind that it is far more important to do your exercises every day, than to do them many times a day. The exercises remind your body to be organized in a particular way, and a couple of reminders seem to be just as effective as a bunch of reminders.

When you do get started on your program, I want you to be hyper-vigilant that you do not aggravate your lower back pain with your rehab efforts. When it appears that the danger of aggravating your pain is no longer an issue, you can schedule an additional routine or two to your day if you so wish. And then do your best to adhere to that schedule. Your body appreciates and thrives on routine.

As you know, the underlying problems that culminated in your body pulling the fire alarm did not occur overnight. Your problems have probably been evolving and accumulating for years, long before you became consciously aware of them. Time now to put that awareness to work by starting on a physical reorganization and re-education program that will lead you to a smarter, healthier and happier body.

This chapter has been all about giving you a perspective on stretching. I think we all expect stretching to be a simple subject, but as you've just read, there's more to it than most people imagine. As you review the exercise progressions in next few chapters, I think you'll find your stretching knowledge helpful.

REMEMBER:

The real secret to effective stretching is to be completely focused on the sensation in the target muscle while you're attempting to stretch it.

CHAPTER 8

The Exercise Progressions

"You can have a ridiculously enormous and complex data set, but if you have the right tools and methodology then it's not a problem."
— AARON KOBLIN

Every exercise in the Alignment First Protocol is designed to encourage a very specific change in your body. And almost everyone who uses this system is pleasantly surprised at how the exercises reveal their own particular challenges. What might be easy for one person will feel difficult for another. It is for this reason that we need ten exercise progressions and not simply ten exercises.

The first five exercise progressions are designed to improve the alignment of your body. They will improve the symmetry of the length and the tone of the big muscles in your hips, thighs and spine. For the majority of us, these are the key issues and muscles underlying chronic lower back pain.

If you are a member of the minority and your pelvic alignment isn't compromised, good for you. You can use the first five exercise progressions to help improve your hip and pelvic mobility. Mobility is a prerequisite in order for you regain healthy, comfortable function in this area of your body.

As outlined earlier in this book, mobility is a prerequisite for all of us. A full range of motion for our major weight-bearing joints is the goal. I mention that progressions seven and eight also consist of mobilizing exercises.

Exercise progressions six, nine and ten add the stability and strength that we need in order to stabilize your new and improved alignment and mobility. Without these exercises, any improvements in function and/or comfort that we might be able to bring about are likely to be short lived. These exercises are the tools you are going to use to begin the process of getting your life back and keeping pain out of it.

Here's a list of the exercise progressions:

1. **Hip Mobility (hip flexion & rotation)**
   A. Knee to Chest Stretch – supine
   B. Hip Lift – supine wall assisted
   C. Hip Crossover – supine
   D. Pigeon Pose
2. **Hip/Knee Mobility (hip flexion & knee extension)**
   A. Hamstring Stretch – supine single leg wall assisted
   B. Hamstring Stretch – supine wall assisted
   C. Hamstring Stretch – seated
   D. Downward Dog
3. **Hip Mobility (hip abduction)**
   A. Inner Thigh Stretch – supine butterfly
   B. Inner Thigh Stretch – supine wall assisted
   C. Groiner
   D. Inner Thigh Stretch – seated
4. **Hip Mobility (hip extension)**
   A. Hip Flexor Stretch – supine
   B. Hip Flexor Stretch – kneeling
   C. Couch Stretch – Position 2
   D. Couch Stretch – Position 3
5. **Hip Mobility (rotation)**
   A. Femur Rotations – supine wall assisted x 20
   B. Femur Rotations – seated x 20
6. **Core Stability**
   A. Modified Dead Bug – with heel drop x 20
   B. Hip Lift
   C. Lower Body Russian Twists x 20
   D. Straight Spine Sit-Ups x 20

7. **Torso/Shoulder Mobility**
   A. Child's Pose
   B. Cats & Dogs x 20
   C. Floor Twist
   D. QL Stretch
8. **Ankle/Foot Mobility and Stability**
   A. Calf Stretch – supine wall assisted
   B. Calf Stretch – standing
   C. Stairway Calf Raises x 20
9. **Multi-Joint Stability**
   A. Alternating Superman
   B. Bird Dog
   C. Forearm Plank
   D. Forearm Side-Plank
10. **Multi-Joint Mobility and Stability**
    A. Squat Stretch – supine wall assisted
    B. Squat Stretch - supported
    C. Wallsit
    D. Deep Squat

You are now equipped with a collection of exercises that you can use to incrementally move your body from chronic pain to pain-free. I know it looks like an awful lot of exercises but don't let first impressions discourage you. It is way less daunting if you think of the Alignment First Protocol as being ten exercises. Because that's the number you will use in your daily routine. Ten. The rest of the exercises are there to accommodate the differing needs of everyone using the protocol. Plus, your mastery of the exercises you use will change over time. Simply focus on ten exercises at a time and chip away at the process to suit your needs. Unless your case is unusually complicated, this system will work for you.

In the next chapter, I will walk you through the least demanding exercise in each of the ten progressions. Chapter 9 is where everyone should begin, for safety's sake. If you are able to perform the full range of motion for one or more of those exercises; and if you can do them in complete comfort and with little effort, feel free to check out the next exercise in the progression, in Chapter 10. If your body says you're able to move to the next exercise in that particular exercise progression, who are you to argue?

As your performance improves, continue your advance through the progression for that exercise. For example, once your body can reliably demonstrate 20 degrees of ankle dorsiflexion in the Supine Calf Stretch, you should switch to the Standing Calf Stretch version of the exercise. Once you can reliably demonstrate 20 degrees of ankle dorsiflexion in that position, you have mastered that piece of the Alignment First Protocol.

For our purposes, there is no greater demand to graduate to. From then on you will simply need to maintain that level of performance. You are not training for the Olympics or the circus and more mobility is not always better.

When you do your daily exercise routine, you should begin each exercise progression wherever you left off, the day before. If your body tells you that you need to regress, or progress, within any exercise progression, that's what you need to do. Listen for the cues from your body and do your best to respect them. Know which exercises are challenging for you and focus on improving those. Be patient. By the time you master the entire protocol, your lower back pain should be a distant and fading memory.

Now it is time to learn the entry level Alignment First Protocol exercises.

CHAPTER 9

Your First Routine

Everything must be made as simple as possible,
but no simpler."
— ALBERT EINSTEIN

The following ten exercises are to be performed in the order they're listed. Each of them is the first exercise in its respective set of exercise progression. Should you be able to easily perform any of the following exercises, please move on to the next exercise in that particular exercise's progression. For example, if 1.A (below) is easy for you, then move on to exercise 1.B. (You'll find exercise 1.B in Chapter 10.)

They all look pretty easy and though each can be completed in a minute or two, you might encounter some challenges. So, start slow. Be gentle. And use your body sensations to reach out and connect with your target muscles. I expect you will enjoy most of these "stretches" and that they will encourage you to adopt the First Alignment Protocol for the good of your lower back.

1.A: Knee to Chest Stretch – supine

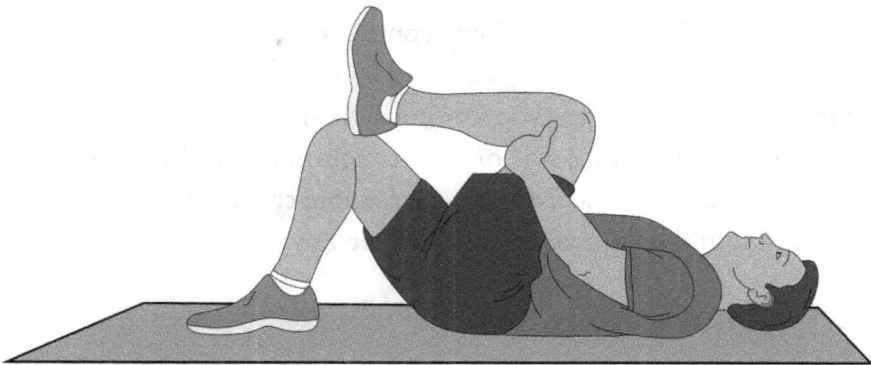

- Get on your back with your knees bent to approximately 90 degrees, your feet 6-8 inches apart and parallel to one another.
- Tighten your abdominal muscles to push your lower back firmly into the floor and hold it stable throughout the exercise.
- Grab hold of your left knee and gently pull it towards the left side of your chest, as far as it will comfortably go. If you feel a comfortable stretch sensation in your left hip, simply hold that stretch for one minute.
- Repeat on the right side.
- Practice your favourite diaphragmatic breathing technique during your stretches. One good option is to slowly count to 7 as you exhale, and again to 7 as you inhale. For most people this will result in a much slower and deeper breathing pattern than they are used to. Breathing like this may be surprisingly challenging initially, especially since you are bracing your lower back at the same time. Don't be discouraged; it will improve with practice.

Modifications

It is rare for anyone to experience aggravated symptoms during this exercise. But it does happen. One modification that I have used successfully, is to place a pool noodle, or a rolled-up hand towel, across and under the lower back. This often creates just enough positional change to eliminate any discomfort. Should this modification make the exercise more comfortable for you, I suggest you consider using the roll/noodle for all of the exercises where you're on your back.

If you find this stretch perfectly comfortable, there is a slight modification you can try before graduating to Exercise 1.B in Chapter 10. Simply straighten the leg you are not holding onto. If you have any shortness in your hip flexor or inner thigh muscles, they will tug on your pelvis. It will immediately be a little more challenging to push your low back into the floor and pull your knee toward your chest.

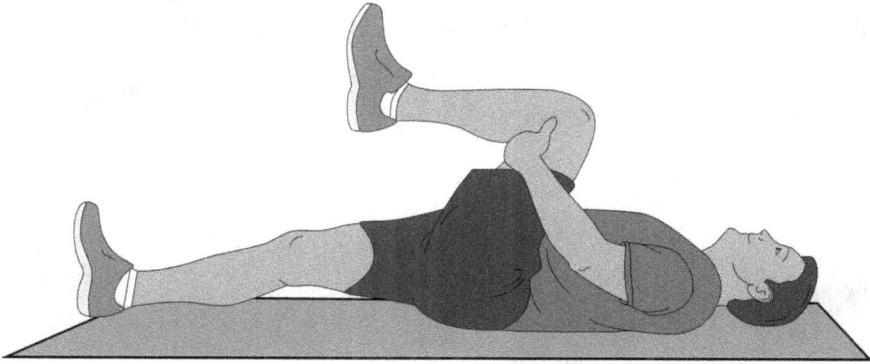

Another variation of this exercise is to pull both knees to your chest, at the same time. This version seems to distribute the stretch more evenly between your glutes and your lower back, when compared to the single leg versions. It can be a useful 'first aid' posture when your lower back is acting up, and most back pain patients are very familiar with it.

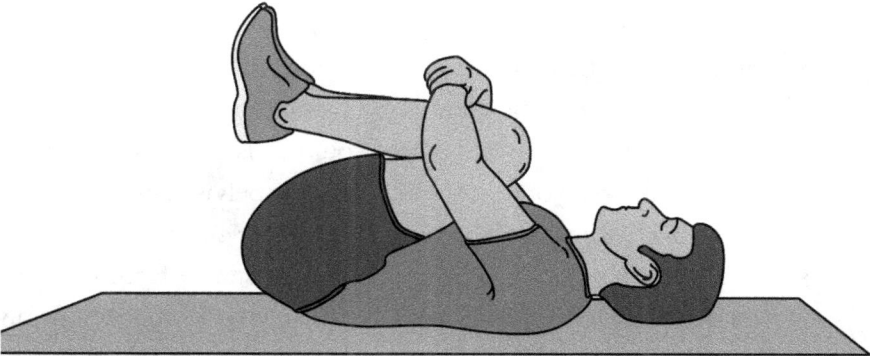

If you have no new pain, or no increased pain, during any of the versions of this exercise, it is time to graduate to Exercise 1.B, Hip Lift – Supine Wall Assisted, in Chapter 10. Look at you! You're making progress already.

2.A: Hamstring Stretch – supine single leg wall assisted

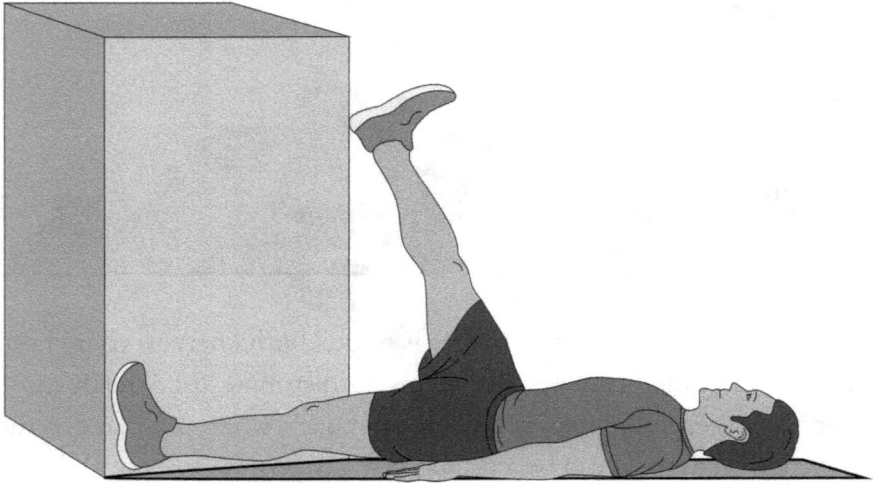

- Get on your back in a doorway and put your right leg up the wall and the left leg flat on the floor.
- Straighten both knees as much as you can and move your right buttock as close to the door frame as you can without letting your knees bend or lifting the back of your pelvis off the floor. If you can't straighten your knees fully or your pelvis is lifting off the floor, that means you need to move further away from the wall.
- Once you have found the appropriate distance from the wall, tighten your abdominal muscles to push your lower back firmly into the floor, and hold it stable there throughout the exercise.
- Make sure that your feet are as perpendicular to the wall and floor as possible. Also, pull your toes towards you as much as you're able.
- Once you are in the proper position, if you feel a stretch sensation in the back of your thigh (hamstrings), take big, slow breaths and relax as best you can. Spend at least one minute in this position, on each side.

Normal hip flexion is considered to be 125 degrees. When lying on your back with your leg up the wall, if your buttock on the side you are stretching comes right up against the door frame, this is only demanding 90 degrees of hip flexion. If you feel a stretch in your lower back, buttocks, hamstrings and/or calves when in this position, it is a clear message from your body that you have some work to do!

It can be next to impossible to reposition the pelvis and/or hips when the hamstring muscles are chronically clenching. Time and time again, however, I have seen how exaggerating the tightness of the core muscles can be used to trick the body into releasing hamstring clenching and immediately improving hip flexion range of motion. This underlines how important and valuable tightening your ab muscles can be to maximize your success in this exercise.

Modifications

If you found this exercise to be pain-producing or pain-increasing, please experiment with the following modifications, in the sequence provided, until you can perform the exercise for one minute:

- Move slightly further away from the wall to lessen the tension in your lower back, inner thigh muscles, glutes and/or hamstrings.
- You can lay a rolled-up hand towel or pool noodle under and across your lower back. This may prevent the exercise from pulling all of the extension curve out of your lower back during this exercise. It may also make it easier for you to push your lower back towards the floor, because the range of motion is less.

You may need one, or a combination, of these modifications to allow you to do the exercise without creating more pain. With diligent practice, you should see gradual improvement in your ability to execute the details of the exercise. This should include improvements in range of motion and comfort. However, if you are able to touch the wall with your buttock on the stretching side; and if you don't feel any stretch sensation in the back of your thigh, you need to graduate to the two-legged version of the stretch (Exercise 2.B Hamstring Stretch – Supine Wall Assisted, in Chapter 10).

3.A: Inner Thigh Stretch – supine butterfly

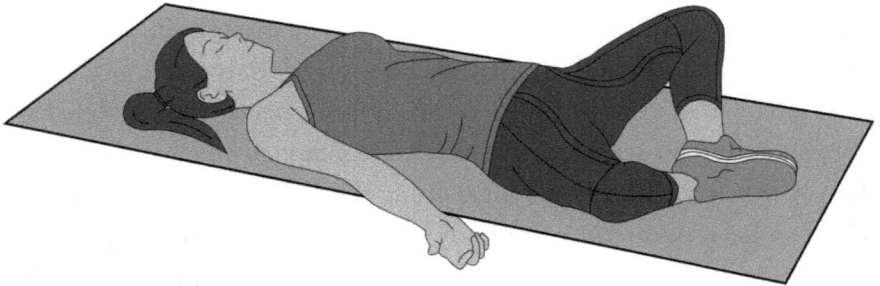

- Lie on your back with your knees bent to approximately 90 degrees, placing your feet and knees together.
- Firmly press your lower back down into the floor and hold it there for the entire stretch.
- Now, put the soles of your feet together and slowly lower your knees towards the floor.

It is critically important to re-educate the inner thigh muscles in any chronic, lower back pain situation. This muscle group plays a significant role as stabilizers during normal physical function. In response to significant levels of misalignment in the lower body, however, they are typically 'turned on' 24/7. Said another way: when your lower body is crooked, your body shortens your inner thigh muscles to brace and stabilize.

Modifications

If you have found this exercise to be pain-producing or pain-increasing, please experiment with the following modifications, in the order given, until you can perform the exercise for one minute:

- Limit how far your legs move apart during the exercise to lessen the tension in your inner thigh muscles. Potentially, this will also lessen the pressure in your hip joints and pelvis. A simple way to do this, is to place a pillow or pillows under your knees. This can create just enough support to remove the discomfort or extra discomfort.

- Experiment by changing how far your feet are from your pelvis. Just by moving your feet closer or further from your pelvis, you can change the angle of pull just enough to make the exercise more comfortable. Conversely, you can position yourself so that your toes contact a wall or heavy piece of furniture. This eliminates your body's need to "hold" your feet and allows you to relax into the stretch more completely. By adding this extra bit of support, you can often improve your experience of, and success with, this exercise.
- If you used a rolled-up hand towel or a pool noodle across your lower back in the first few exercises, you will likely need the towel/noodle during this exercise as well.

If this exercise has not caused pain or an increase of existing pain, you're off to a good start!

If you can already separate your legs 90 degrees (normal hip abduction is considered to be 45 degrees per side), it is time to graduate to the straight legged, wall assisted version of this exercise (Exercise 3.B, Inner Thigh Stretch – Supine Wall Assisted, in Chapter 10).

4.A: Hip Flexor Stretch – supine

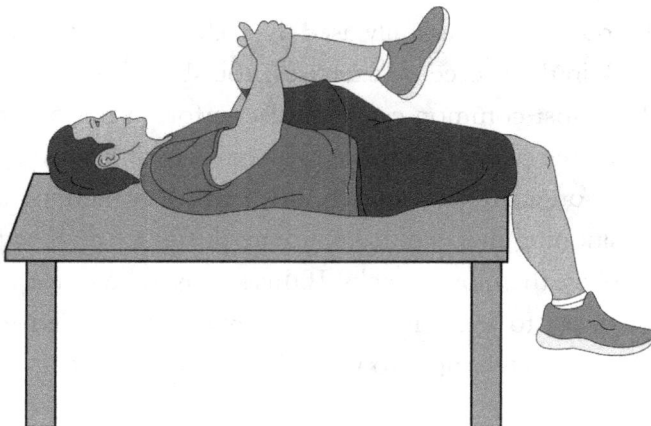

- Lie on your back on a bench, table or even your bed. You need to be near the edge of the surface you are on, but make sure it feels stable enough for you to relax.
- Starting with both knees bent and legs together, use your hands to grab both thighs and pull them towards your chest as far as they will comfortably go.
- Try to push your lower back down into the surface you are lying on and hold it there, for the duration of the exercise.
- Continue to hold your left knee as close to your chest as you can and release your hold on the right thigh. Lower your right leg, over the side of the surface you are lying on. Let it hang freely in the air. Don't pull the leg towards the floor. Just let gravity do its thing.
- Breathe deeply and try to feel a stretch sensation in the front of your right hip/thigh. It is the hip you are NOT pulling on that we are stretching.
- After one minute, pull your right thigh back up to your chest and slowly lower your left leg and foot over the side and repeat the stretch.

Modifications

- If you've found this exercise to be pain-producing or pain-increasing, try using a little less force when pulling your thigh towards your chest.
- If you have successfully used the roll/noodle under your lower back in the preceding exercises, you should try it here as well.
- The most common cause of discomfort in this stretch occurs when the person is unable to stabilize their lumbar spine. This is a non-aggressive stretch, but there is something about the positioning that can make it quite difficult for some people to stabilize their lower backs. If this seems to be so for you, please graduate to Exercise 4.B. You may find the Kneeling Hip Flexor Stretch more to your liking and comfort.

- If, on the other hand, you have no pain and are able to get a full range of motion in hip extension (40 degrees) during this exercise, you also need to graduate to Exercise 4.B in Chapter 10.

5.A: Femur Rotations x 20 – supine wall assisted

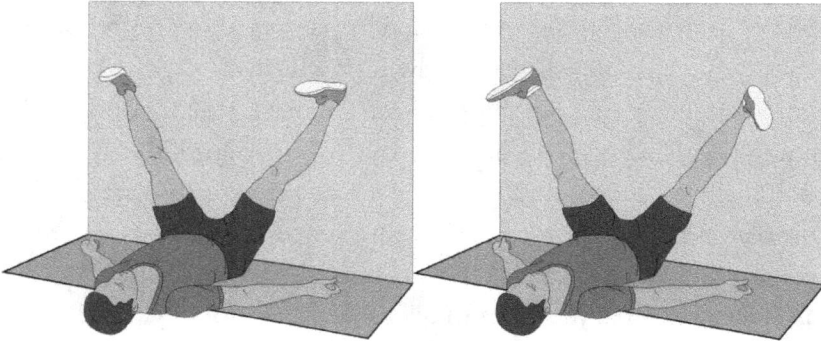

- This exercise begins with you on your back, legs up the wall, with your body as close to the wall as you can be and still keep your knees straight.
- Keeping your knees fully extended and your toes pulled towards you (ankles dorsiflexed), move your feet approximately one yard/one meter apart (the distance doesn't have to be exact).
- While maintaining all of the positional elements mentioned, rotate your knees/feet towards one another and then away from one another, at a slow, steady pace. Pause slightly at the end of each movement.
- Repeat 20 times.

This exercise is all about addressing rotational mobility of the hip joints. It is important to understand that this exercise is not about strengthening these muscles. At this stage of the process, we are really only concerned about alignment (first) and mobility (second).

Normal "external" range of motion is considered to be 45 degrees. For "internal" rotation, normal range is 40 degrees. If you perceive that your range of movement is obviously less than 40-45 degrees in these movements, then that is something to keep an eye on. Because opinions can vary over what "normal" range of motion numbers should be, it may be tempting to ignore the numbers I am using here. But here's the thing: any large discrepancy, between the range of motion numbers I am using and what you see in your own body, is a cause for concern.

Please pay attention to your body's ability to achieve the range of motion I list for specific exercises. And be particularly wary of differences between the two sides of your body. If you have 40 degrees of external rotation in both of your hips, I don't expect you to obsess about training them to get to 45 degrees. But if your right hip can only give you 20 degrees and your left can't give you any external rotation, that's cause for concern. Such right/left differences in mobility are reliable predictors of future pain and dysfunction.

Imbalances signal the types of alignment and mobility problems that prevent your body from functioning in a safe and comfortable manner. It's important to identify these imbalances and work on eliminating them. I'm not saying that you need to get out a laser measuring device, but if it helps to refresh your 'mind's eye protractor' let's do it. You know what a ninety-degree angle looks like. Half of that is 45 degrees (diagonal line in a square). If, in your mind's eye, you can cut that triangle in half two more times (22.5 degrees and 11.25 degrees) and be even remotely in the right ballpark, you can handle the geometry needed to manage your body through this process.

Modifications

If this exercise causes you pain or increases your pain, please experiment with the following modifications, in the sequence provided. Your objective is to perform the exercise without causing or increasing pain:

- Experiment with holding your legs either a little further apart or a little closer together. By simply changing the amount of tension in your hip joints and pelvis, this may help.
- Move slightly further away from the wall to lessen the tension in your lower back.

- If you used the towel/noodle under your lower back for the preceding exercises, you might want to keep using it for all of the exercises that have you on your back.

If this exercise has not caused pain or increased existing pain, and if you can already perform this exercise through a full range of motion, it's time to graduate to a seated version of this same exercise (exercise 5.B, called Femur Rotations - Seated Wall Assisted, in Chapter 10).

6.A: Modified Dead Bug (with heel drop) x 10 each side

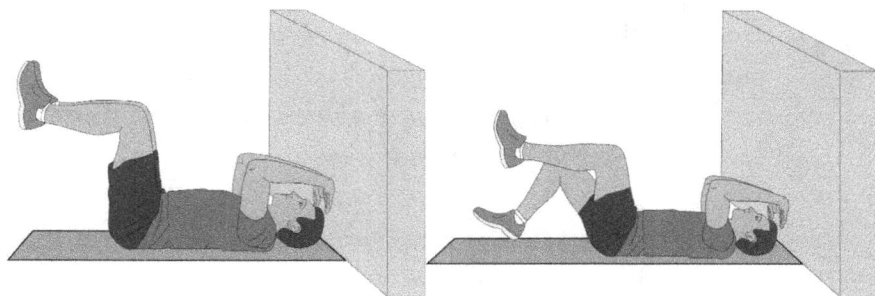

- Lie on your back with your head a couple inches from a wall, with your knees bent and feet flat on the floor.
- Place your hands on the wall with your fingers pointing towards the floor, your elbows high and shoulder width apart. Push your hands firmly into the wall. Remember, your body likes stability, so use your hands to stabilize it.
- Lift your feet off the floor so your thighs are vertical, and your lower legs are parallel to the floor.
- Bend your toes towards both knees and hold them there.
- Try to tighten your core muscles and flatten your lower back into the floor, holding it there for the duration of the exercise.
- Slowly lower your right heel towards the floor, without changing the amount of bend at your knee, as far as you can without allowing your lower back to come up off the floor.

- As long as you are not creating new pain or aggravating existing pain, lift the right foot back to the starting position and repeat, a total of ten times.
- Don't forget to breathe! Controlling your breathing, at a rate of 7 seconds per inhalation and 7 seconds per exhalation, may make the exercise seem harder initially, but your efforts will pay off in the end.
- Repeat the exercise with your left foot, ten times as well.

Modifications

- If you've found this exercise to be pain-producing or pain-increasing, please try again. But this time, try using a smaller range of motion and maybe, don't do as many repetitions.
- If you've needed a roll under your lower back during the earlier exercises, you will likely need it here as well.

This is the first exercise, in this set of progressions, designed to stimulate muscular activity for the sake of stability. Its primary goal is to neither align nor mobilize. You are now at the point in your routine where you're beginning to ask your new and improved alignment to start pulling its own weight, so to say.

Ideally, you can perform the prescribed movement through a full range of motion (from vertical thigh to foot touching the floor and back again). And do so without pain or increased pain. But it's not a deal breaker if you can't. In fact, I want to emphasize that it's far more important you avoid creating or aggravating back pain, than it is to set a personal record for completing an exercise. Go easy. Respect your symptoms. Practice what your body will allow. And trust in the process. Work up to 20 reps on each side.

When you can do this exercise without pain, it's time to move on to Exercise 6.B, called Hip Lift in Chapter 10.

7.A: Child's Pose

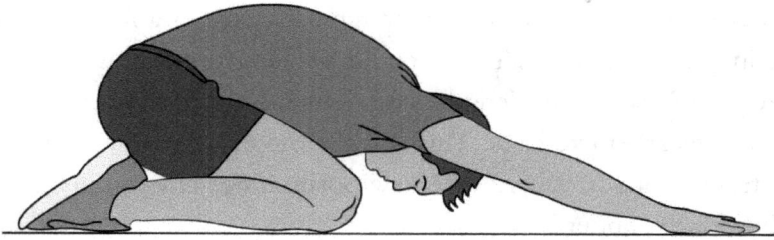

- Get down on your hands and knees, then sit back with your buttocks towards your heels.
- Depending upon what is most comfortable, you can go down onto your forearms, crossing one forearm over the other and then resting your forehead on the top of your topmost forearm. If you can do that easily, try placing your arms back beside your body with your palms up. Or reach forward on the floor with your palms down. If you choose either of these latter two positions, rest your forehead on the floor.
- Note: if you experience any discomfort in your neck or back whatsoever, please rest your head on your forearms instead of the floor.
- It can be particularly helpful to focus breathing into your lower abdomen while in this posture. It seems to be an effective way to maximize the amount of lower back relaxation during this exercise.

This is the first exercise in the routine that does not have you on your back, with your lower back supported by the floor. The other exercises have helped to prepare your body to safely and comfortably manage your spinal position without direct support from the floor.

For many people with back pain, this exercise is initially as much a front of thigh stretch (quadriceps) as anything else. It will also reveal if the person doing the exercise is very short or tight through the front of their ankles and lower legs. In such cases, it is difficult and uncomfortable to try to relax the ankles towards the floor.

You will probably feel a mild stretch sensation or a feeling of tightness in your lower back. This exercise will almost certainly add slightly more straightening and lengthening demand to your lower back than any of the earlier exercises. This is really the first exercise in the series that truly begins to "share" the new positioning achieved in the lower body with the upper body.

Modifications

If you found this exercise to be pain-producing or pain-increasing, please experiment with the following modifications, in the following sequence, until you can perform the exercise for one minute:

- Kneel on a soft surface to protect your knees, such as your bed or an exercise mat.
- Put a rolled-up towel or pool noodle under your ankles to lessen the stretch tension in the front of your lower legs/ankles.
- Put a pillow (or more than one) behind your knees to limit knee flexion and lessen the stretch tension in your knees.
- Put a pillow (or more than one) between the tops of your thighs and your abdomen to limit hip flexion and lessen the stretch tension in your hips/pelvis.
- Use a pillow (or more than one) under your forearms to limit hip and lumbar flexion, lessening the stretch tension in your hips, pelvis and lower back.

If you are able to do the version of this exercise where you are reaching forward along the floor, palms down and forehead touching the floor; and if you have little or no stretch sensation in that position; and if it has not created pain or increased existing pain; you are ready to graduate to exercise 7.B, called Cats & Dogs in Chapter 10.

8.A: Calf Stretch – supine wall assisted

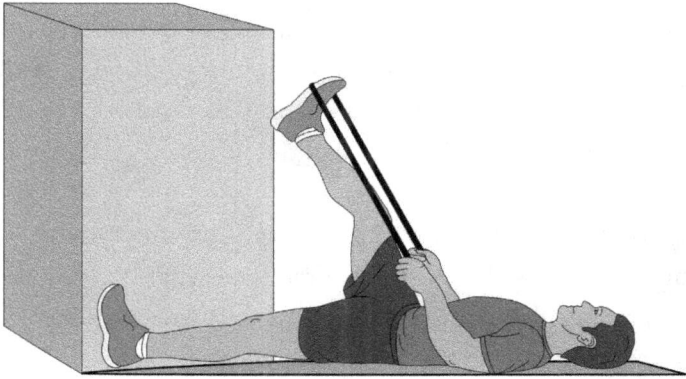

- Start this exercise on your back, with your legs up the wall, and your buttocks as close to the wall as you can go while keeping your knees completely straight.
- If you can't straighten your knees fully or your pelvis is suspended up off the floor, that means you need to move further away from the wall.
- Put your feet together and loop a rope, yoga strap or exercise band around the balls of both feet. It's important that you are not catching only your toes.
- Gently pull the balls of your feet towards you, without creating pain in your lower back.
- If you find that you have to pull really hard to feel stretch in your feet and calves, try stretching one leg at a time. It may be more comfortable and more efficient to do it that way.
- Take big, slow breaths, relaxing as best you can. Spend at least a minute in this position (that's one minute for each leg if you are doing them one at a time).

Shin splints, plantar fasciitis and bunions are some of the most obvious ailments directly related to short calf muscles. Walking, running, jumping and squatting mechanics all become compromised and problematic if you don't maintain adequate mobility in your ankles and feet.

Modifications

- If you found this exercise to be pain-producing or pain-increasing, you should move further away from the wall. That will decrease the amount of tension in your lower body.
- You can also try simply pulling less hard on your foot/feet.
- Try bending your knee(s) slightly.

If you don't experience any aggravating symptoms doing this exercise, congratulations! There is quite a range of what is considered to be normal full range of motion, when it comes to ankle mobility. However, most references I've seen suggest 20 degrees of dorsiflexion (pointing your toes at your knees) and 45 degrees of plantar flexion (pointing your toes away from your knees).

We are seeking to improve dorsiflexion with this exercise. If you can already get 20 degrees of dorsiflexion in this exercise, you should progress to the standing version of this exercise (8.B in Chapter 10). Note: when you perform the Standing Calf Stretch for the first time, if you can immediately demonstrate 20 degrees of dorsiflexion, promote yourself to exercise 8.C, Standing Calf Raises. This is because too much mobility can be just as problematic as not enough, especially if you don't have the strength and stability to control it. So, whatever you do, don't spend a bunch of time on this exercise, unless you are having a tough time achieving your range of motion goal.

9.A: Alternating Superman

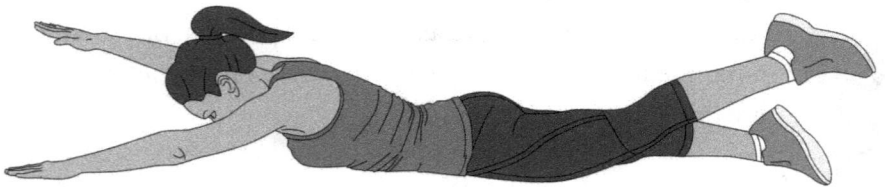

- Go flat on your stomach (prone), with your legs straight and relaxed and your arms on the floor and loosely stretched out in front of you, hands approximately shoulder width apart.
- Keep your nose pointed directly at the floor throughout the exercise.
- Keeping your core muscles as tight as you can, and your knees and elbow straight, slowly lift your right hand and left foot up off the floor slightly and hold them there.
- The goal during this exercise is to get your right hand and left foot up off the floor *as far as comfortably possible, but it is critical that you do not push this exercise into pain.*
- Although the goal is to hold this position for 30 seconds on each side, you may have to break that 30 seconds into smaller chunks. It is not unusual, in fact, for lower back pain patients to begin with holds lasting less than ten seconds.
- You are obtaining considerable support and stability from the floor in this exercise. Do not waste that support by lifting your foot and knee off the floor like an Olympic gymnast, unless you can do so with 100% comfort. And by the way, if it feels considerably better to keep both feet on the floor when you do this exercise for the first few times, feel free to keep them there.

Modifications

If you found this exercise to be pain-producing or pain-increasing, please experiment with the following modifications, in the order given, until you can perform the exercise for 30 seconds straight, on each side:

- My favorite modification of this exercise is to put a pillow under the abdomen. This helps to increase abdominal pressure, making bracing easier. It also decreases the amount of lower back extension.
- Another way to reduce the demand is to leave the foot on the extending hip side on the floor to add stability. Delay lifting

the foot up off the floor until you can do so without creating pain in your lower back.

- Trying to lift your arm too high can quickly exceed the amount of shoulder and spine mobility that your body is willing to give you, at this stage. This can force you into pain, awkward positions or both. So please, don't do it.

- In the event of uncomfortable neck irritation, you may have to keep your forehead on the floor, typically supported by a pillow or rolled up exercise mat. Another strategy is to put one of your hands under your forehead instead of reaching ahead with it. I've seen it work well using the resting hand. In cases where the neck is less symptomatic, we have used the lifting hand instead. If you feel that your neck needs support during this exercise, experiment with these three options and use the one most comfortable for you.

- If you a hold your limbs up off the floor for 30 seconds with little effort and no pain or no increasing pain, move on to the Bird Dog, exercise 9.B in Chapter 10.

10.A: Squat Stretch – supine wall assisted

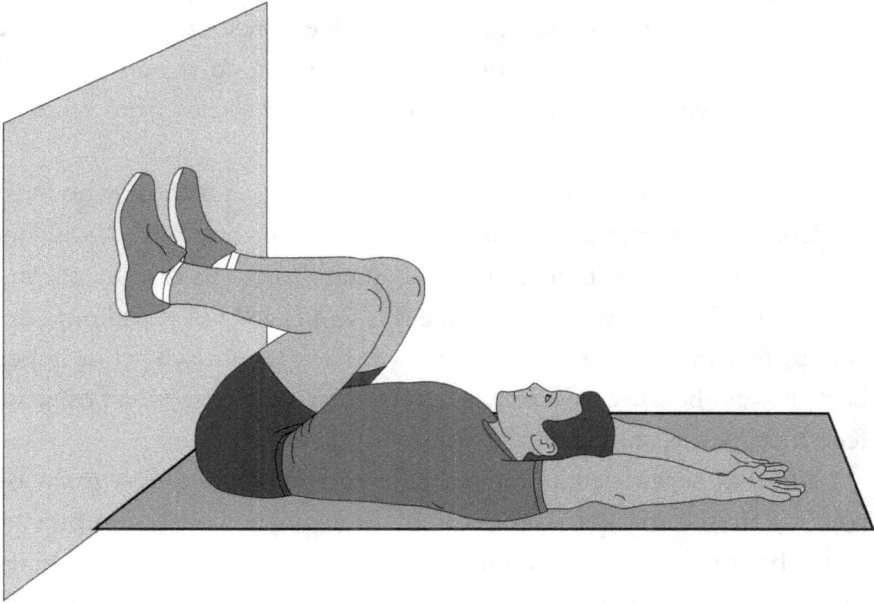

- Lie on your back with your legs up the wall, your knees bent and your feet together.
- We want your buttocks as close to the wall as possible, so use carpet or an exercise mat to prevent you from sliding away from the wall.
- Put the soles of your feet against the wall, as parallel to each other as possible.
- Make you lower legs as close to parallel to the floor as possible.
- Pull your feet as far apart from one another as possible, while keeping them vertically aligned and your lower legs still parallel to the floor.
- While maintaining the other positional elements, pull your knees as far apart as possible.
- Try to tighten your abdominal muscles and firmly push your lower back down into the floor, holding it there for the duration of the exercise.

- Last but not least, put your hands overhead, palms up, with elbows straight. Move your elbows as close to your ears as you can, as long as your forearms are able to rest on the floor. You do not want to let you your arms dangle in the air: that will prevent your shoulder, chest and back muscles from relaxing into the stretch.

This exercise is unlikely to cause positional stress for those who have no problem with range of motion restrictions in their hips, shoulders or spine. By the same token, this book in unlikely to be read by anyone resembling that description. So, take this as a heads up: you should expect to feel stretch tension in your lower back (and maybe your upper back as well) because this exercise exerts a straightening effect on your feet, hips, pelvis, shoulders and spine.

I add that because this exercise tends to add tension to so many of your big muscle groups and because it also simultaneously compresses your abdomen, it is important for you to focus on your breathing. Breathe as deeply as possible and while you're at it, please don't allow your ribcage to flare upward.

I know that I have recommended you hold your exercise poses for one minute, but feel free to linger in this one a little while longer. Most of the exercises so far, have helped prepare your body to be better in this exercise. Still and all, most people are surprised by how much stretch tension they can feel throughout their body in this position.

This exercise really connects the dots for many lower back pain sufferers. That's because it often reveals positional/tension imbalances in a whole-body context that isn't experienced when exercising your body parts in the piecemeal fashion we've been doing so far. A little extra time spent reorganizing the body with this particular exercise is time very well spent.

Modifications

If you found this exercise to be pain-producing or pain-increasing, please experiment with the following modifications, in the order given, until you can perform the exercise for one minute:

- Move slightly further away from the wall to lessen the tension in your hips and lower back.
- Experiment with not pushing your knees so far apart.
- Try holding your feet a little closer together to decrease the amount of tension in your hips.
- If you used the rolled-up towel/pool noodle across your lower back in earlier supine exercises, you will quite likely need it for this one as well.
- Go easy on where and how you place your arms. If you have enough flexion in your thoracic spine and/or enough dysfunctional tension in your shoulders, you trying to force your arms up beside your ears could create unwanted extension pressure in your lower back. Try putting your arms out at right angles to your torso and see if that lessens your back discomfort. As your condition improves, you can gradually raise your arms toward the overhead position without recreating lower back pain.

If you can get your buttocks up to the wall and if you are not feeling much of a stretch anywhere during this exercise, you have mastered it. You're now ready to graduate to exercise 10.B in Chapter 10.

This chapter has introduced you to the least demanding exercise in each of the ten exercise progressions. You've probably found one or two that stand out as being either particularly tough or particularly easy. That's good. That's normal.

As you work with these exercises, your body will signal when it's time to move on to the next higher degree of demand. You'll get the signal when you realize that an exercise is no longer challenging your body in any way. That's your cue to move to the next exercise in that particular set of exercise progressions.

In those exercises where you're training one side of your body at a time, you may find one side to be less mobile than the other. When this happens, apply twice as much training to the restricted side until the two sides become equal. (Please base your assessment on mobility; not "tightness". As a yardstick, tightness can be deceiving.) For example, if during the Hip

Flexor Stretch you find that your right side is significantly less mobile than your left, simply repeat the stretch a second time on the right. This simple modification to your routine can make all the difference in the world.

If you have already found an exercise (or two) to be particularly challenging, that is a clear sign that you have found an issue that needs to be corrected. Try to be patient with these particular exercises and with your body. Your persistent, gentle insistence will allow your body no alternative but to gradually improve its performance of these exercises. It may feel like a small victory but over time, they add up big improvements.

As already noted, the next chapter contains more exercise instructions. Use them to help you measure, guide and maintain your progress toward your target: a life without the constraints of chronic lower back pain.

CHAPTER 10

The Rest of the Exercises

"A huge body of research has shown that small wins have enormous power, an influence disproportionate to the accomplishments of the victories themselves."
— CHARLES DUHIGG

As we move further into the exercise progressions, I am reminded of the line, "Everything is hard before it is easy." It's so appropriate for just about every process I've encountered, including the Alignment First Protocol. Every one of its exercises looks and sounds more "hard" than it turns out to be.

And I know, some of the exercise instructions seem pretty complicated, too. If they're over-explained, that's on me. But I want you to do them properly and more importantly, to be safe when doing them. So, as you encounter a new exercise, please humour me and my cautious nature. Take the time to follow the step-by-step directions. And if you don't mind, try to turn the volume up on your body-sensing instincts and intuitions. You really can feel your way into and out of these exercises, you'll see.

("Everything is hard before it is easy." is ascribed to the German author, J.W. Goethe.)

1.B: Hip Lift – wall assisted

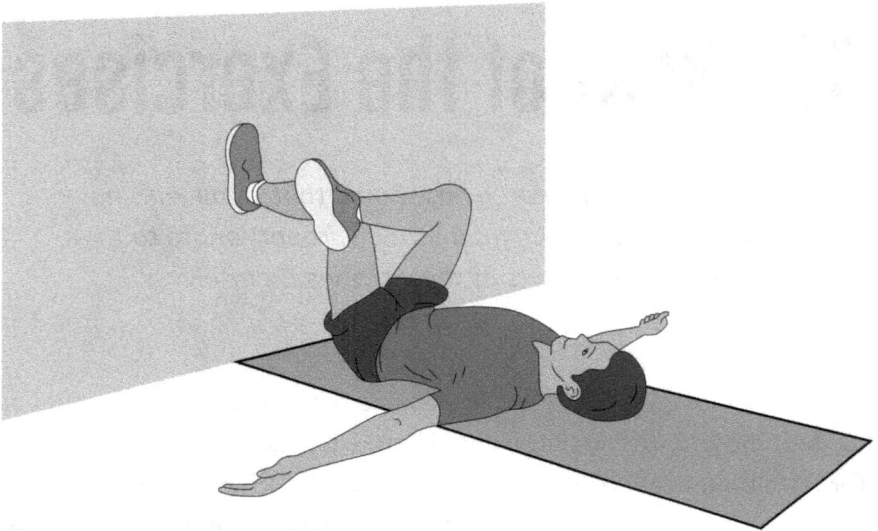

- Get on your back with the soles of your feet flat on the wall.
- Find the proper distance from the wall so that your hips and knees are flexed to 90 degrees.
- Keeping your left foot vertical on the wall, place the outside of your right ankle on top of your left thigh, just above your knee.
- If this position causes you pain or lifts the back of your pelvis off the floor, move away from the wall until those problems disappear. If you feel no stretch sensation in your right buttock, you need to move closer to the wall until you do feel a stretch.
- Once you feel a stretch sensation in your right buttock, while having the back of your pelvis on the floor and without experiencing increasing pain, you're in the correct position.
- After one minute in this position, repeat the same stretch on the opposite side. You may have to adjust your positioning, either closer to or further from the wall, to feel the appropriate amount of stretch in your buttock muscles. Be alert for a tightness imbalance between your two hips.

This exercise helps you to minimize the typical muscle imbalances that often cause or perpetuate pelvic and/or hip alignment problems.

Because you are in what's called "the Figure 4 Position" (it looks like the number 4) for this exercise, any mobility restriction will almost certainly be caused by shortness in the soft tissues of the opposite buttock and/or lower back. It is not due to anything inherently wrong with the "lifting" hip. (Just to be clear, the lifting hip in the illustration is the one on the LEFT.) Remember, full range of motion in hip flexion is considered to be 125 degrees.

It's quite common to experience range of motion differences between the two hips in this exercise. So, it is important to be on the lookout for such imbalances and then work on correcting them. A sound strategy for this exercise, is to double the amount of stretching you do, on the more restricted side. For example, if you found that your right hip was tighter and less mobile than the left, you should stretch your right buttock, then the left and finally, stretch the right buttock a second time.

This illustrates the concept of using an "imbalanced corrective routine" to bring about balance in an imbalanced body. If you stretch both sides equally, you might achieve some lengthening of the target muscle(s), but you will likely have little success realigning the skeleton. It is essential to understand that lengthening the soft tissues without normalizing the bony alignment is dangerously close to a waste of time.

Modifications

If you found this exercise to be pain-producing or pain-increasing, please experiment with the following modifications, in the order given, until you can perform the exercise for one minute:

- Move slightly further away from the wall to lessen the tension in your hip and lower back.
- Place a rolled-up hand towel or pool noodle across your lower back. This will prevent the exercise from pulling all of the extension curve out of your lower back during the exercise.

If you have your hips virtually on the wall and are not feeling much of a stretch in your buttock, this exercise has nothing more to offer you. Move on to the next exercise in the progression, 1.C, Hip Crossover.

1.C: Hip Crossover

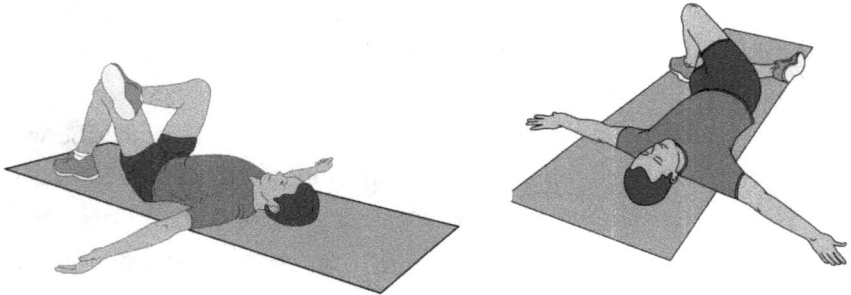

- Get on your back with your knees bent to approximately 90 degrees and the soles of your feet flat on the floor.
- Place the outside of your right ankle on top of your left thigh just above your knee.
- Put your hands at shoulder height on the floor with palms down, to stabilize your upper body.
- Your upper body should be passive and relaxed, with your head turned to neither side.
- Keeping your ankle "glued" in place to your thigh, rotate your lower body (from the hips down) to the left. A full range of motion in this movement will allow you to put the outside of your left thigh and sole of right foot flat on the floor.
- Once your lower body is rotated as far as it can go, using only your hip muscles, push your right knee as far away from your head as far as it will go. You should be able to stand that thigh up to "vertical" (90 degrees of hip abduction) or slightly beyond. Continue to gently maintain that position for one minute.
- Repeat the stretch on the other side for one minute.

This exercise is all about producing a nonaggressive stretch in your lower back, hips and thighs. As always, be alert for imbalances between the two sides of your body in terms of mobility, "tightness" and discomfort. If you find that you are noticeably less mobile on one side, you would not be wrong to double up your efforts on that side (i.e. stretch left, then right and finally, stretch the left side, once again). Eventually, this will help bring both sides of your body into balance.

Modifications

- If, when trying to rotate all the way over to the floor, you feel pain, in either your lower back or your hip, try placing a pillow or another suitable object in the path of your thigh/foot to restrict your range of motion. This will usually allow you to still feel a stretch but eliminate the pain from the exercise.

If you can rotate your lower body all the way over to the floor without contorting your upper body into weird positions; and if you are not feeling much of a stretch in your lower back, hips or thighs, you have mastered this exercise. It's time to move on to the next exercise in the progression, 1.D, Pigeon Pose.

1.D: Pigeon Pose

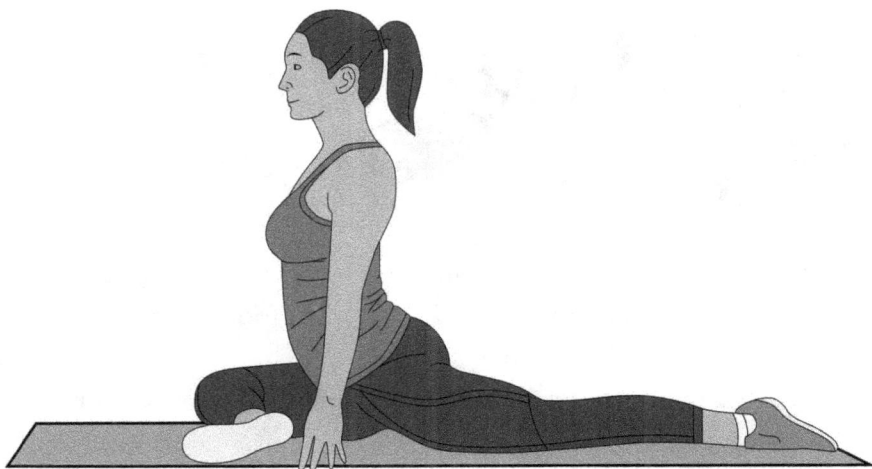

- I realize yoga purists will cringe at this non-traditional entry into the Proud Pigeon Pose, but that's okay.
- Start on your hands and knees, and while bringing your right knee forward, try to place it in the midline of your body, under your abdomen.
- Momentarily lift your left knee off the floor so you can cross your legs, sliding your right knee in front of your left knee, and placing your right foot to the left of your left hip. Once the right foot is on the left side of your body, put the left knee back on the floor.
- Slide your left leg backward along the floor and lower your pelvis towards the floor as far as you can.
- Note: I find that most people need to do the Sleeping Pigeon variation to begin with. (See this pose in the illustration below.) For this 'sleeping' pose, lower your upper body forward/toward (or onto) your right thigh. If you're unable to get all the way down to your thigh, you can support your upper body on your forearms. This can add a very healthy lower back stretch into this exercise.

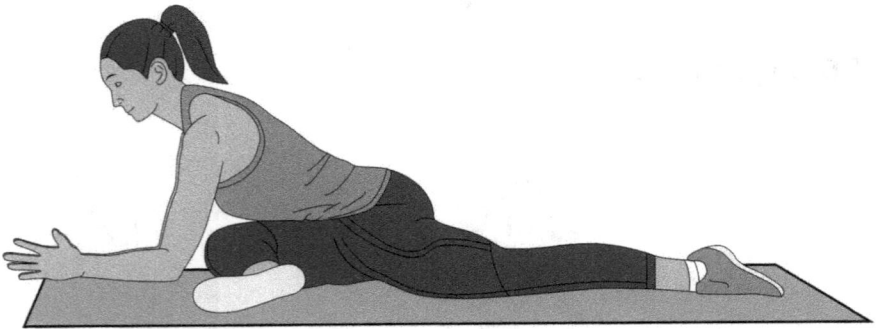

- If you feel that you can add more stretch demand, gently pull your lead foot further forward (e.g. right foot towards left elbow in the illustration above).
- Relax into this position for one minute, then switch sides and repeat.

Modifications

If this exercise caused you pain or increased your pain, please experiment with the following modifications, in the order given, until you can perform the exercise for one minute:

- Perform the exercise on a softer surface, such as your bed or an exercise mat.
- Don't force your legs so far apart.
- Note: If the Pigeon exercise creates or increases knee pain, you should try the Figure 4 Glute Stretch (illustrated below) instead. This exercise begins in exactly the same way as the 1.B Hip Lift (wall assisted). Once in that position, use your hands to grab the upright thigh and pull it toward your chest, until you feel a stretch sensation in your buttock and/or lower back. Hold it for a minute and then repeat with the other thigh. Do your best to keep your head and upper back on the floor.

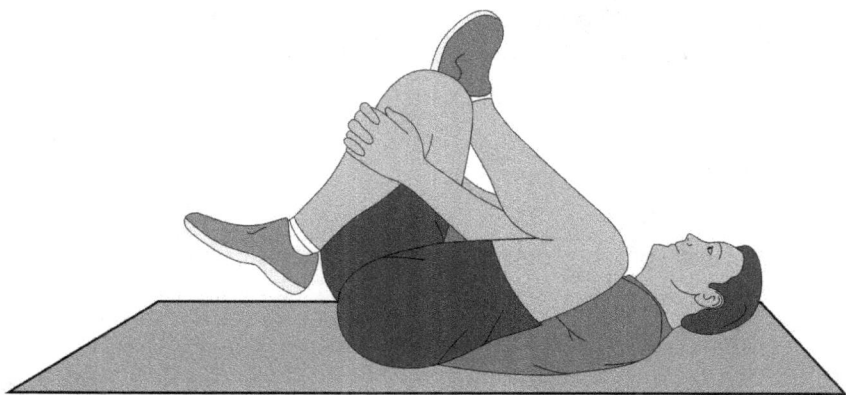

And now, back to the Pigeon Pose. If you can put your chest down onto your thigh when doing Sleeping Pigeon (on each side); and if you can also do the upright torso version (Proud Pigeon) of the exercise without feeling much of a stretch in your lower back or buttocks, you've mastered it! In doing so, you've also mastered the entire first exercise progression. This is a benchmark for you because the Pigeon Pose is the maintenance exercise for this exercise progression. Please continue practicing and perfecting your execution of this exercise.

2.B: Hamstring Stretch – wall assisted

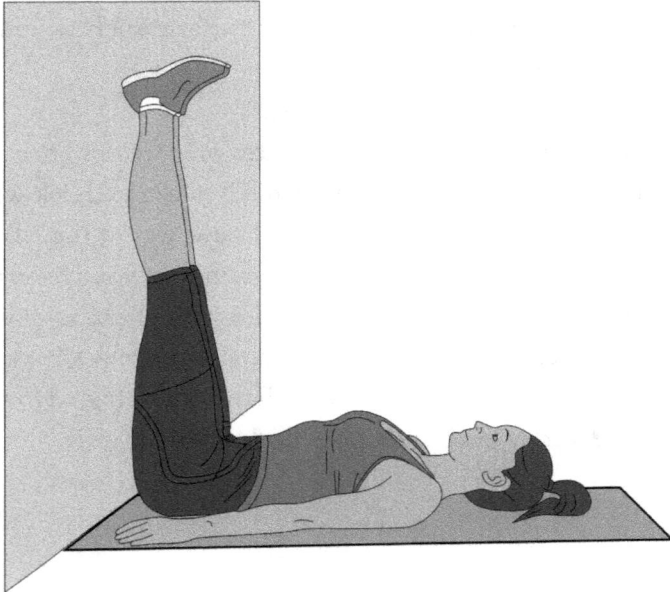

- Get on your back with your legs up the wall and your feet together.
- Move your buttocks as close to the wall as possible, without letting your knees bend or lifting the back of your pelvis off the floor. If you can't straighten your knees fully, or your pelvis does lift off the floor, you'll need to move further away from the wall.
- If your buttocks are against the wall and you feel a stretch sensation in the back of your thighs (hamstrings) with no pain in your back, that is perfect. Now just practice your deep breathing exercise while you remain in this position for one minute.

The mechanics of this exercise will tend to promote straightening and decompression of your lumbar spine by gently stretching the soft tissues of the lower back (as well as those of the glutes and hamstrings).

Modifications

If you found this exercise to be pain-producing or pain-increasing, please experiment with the following modifications, in the order given, until you can perform the exercise for one minute:

- Move slightly further away from the wall to lessen the tension in your lower back, glutes and/or hamstrings.
- Note: for some people, moving away from the wall is not the ideal modification. These people receive more benefit by allowing a slight bend in the knees to leak away the tension that is causing their discomfort.
- If you used a rolled-up hand towel or a pool noodle across your lower back for previous exercises, you should probably do it during this exercise as well. This will avoid pulling all of the extension curve out of your lower back.

If you don't feel much stretch with your legs resting on the wall, you could use a rope/strap/band to pull your legs away from the wall. This could enhance the stretch. However, the better option is to graduate to a Seated Hamstring Stretch (2.C below). This version of the exercise allows you to continue working on lengthening your hamstring muscles, while simultaneously enhancing your ability to stabilize your core with your torso in an upright position.

2.C: Hamstring Stretch – seated

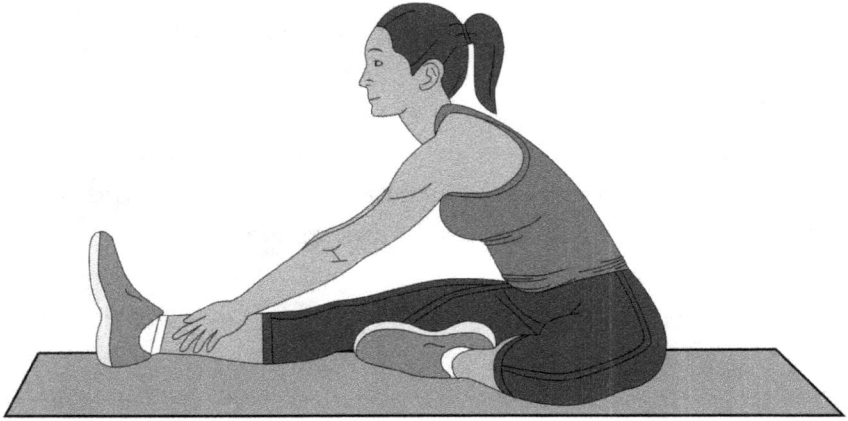

- Sit with your right leg out in front of you and the bottom of your left foot resting against the inside of your right thigh.
- Pull the toes of your right foot towards you and straighten your right knee as much as you're able.
- Tighten your core muscles and keep your spine as rigid as possible while you slowly lower your chest towards your outstretched leg. Move as far as necessary to feel a stretch in your hamstrings, without creating pain in your lower back.
- Take big, slow breaths and spend a minute in this position per side. It is particularly important for your long-term success that you prevent your back from rounding during this and other upright torso exercises. So please, keep your spine as straight and rigid as possible.

Modifications

If you found this exercise to be pain-producing or pain-increasing, the most like problem is related to an inability to stabilize your spine.

- You might eliminate the irritation by simply not leaning so far forward or by using less force to move forward. If that change doesn't minimize the irritation, you should go back to Exercise 2.B, Hamstring

Stretch – wall assisted, for the time being. Your body may need more time for the combined effects of the other exercises, to improve it sufficiently to stabilize your lumbar spine (when in an upright posture). If that's the case, simply retry the seated hamstring stretch, once a week, until you can do it comfortably. As you diligently practice the exercises of the protocol, you will gradually move towards your goal of having a pain-free lower back.

- When you can keep your spine straight and rigid, while you lean forward far enough to reach your foot with both hands (I realize this is a very arbitrary goal, but it works), any pain problems in your lower back probably have little to do with hamstring shortness. At this point, it is much more likely that your need for spinal stability is far greater than your need for increased hamstring length. Please graduate to the next exercise.

2.D: Downward Dog

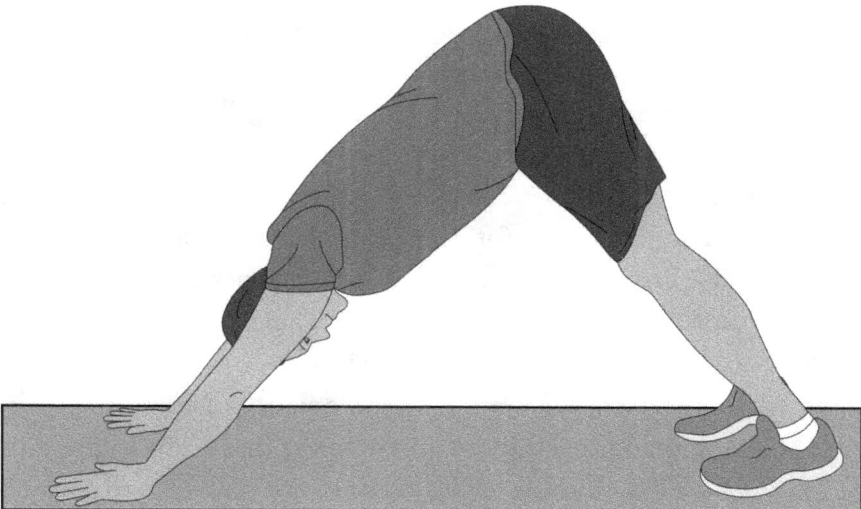

- Start on your hands and knees, with your arms and thighs as perpendicular to the floor as possible. Your hands should be shoulder-width apart and your feet should be hip-width apart, with your fingers and feet pointed straight ahead of you.

- Tuck your toes under and push up onto your feet. Don't move your hands or feet from these positions.
- Try to make your body create two straight lines, one from your hips down to your heels; and the other going down from your hips to your hands. You should look like an upside-down V.
- Straighten your spine, knees and elbows as much as you can. Try to get your heels down onto the floor.
- Practice your deep, slow breathing while you simultaneously hold your core muscles tight. This skill by itself is a significant accomplishment, and if you can do it with ease you are doing very well.

Modifications

If you found this exercise to be pain-producing or pain-increasing, please experiment with the following modifications, in the order given, until you can perform the exercise for one minute:

- As mentioned, because you have come so far in the protocol, any pain produced during this exercise is unlikely to be caused by hamstring shortening. It is more likely due to an inability to stabilize your lower back sufficiently. Therefore, your first modification should be to double down on your efforts to tighten your core. First, try forcefully expelling all the air in your lungs and aggressively squeezing your core muscles. And then experiment by trying the opposite. Try taking a big breath in and holding it, while you aggressively brace your muscles around that held breath. Do either of these strategies lessen your pain?
- Try moving your hands forward, away from your feet slightly. This will decrease the demand for your hip to flex and possibly, allow you to lessen the excessive tension in your lower back, glutes and/or hamstrings.
- Simply bend your knees slightly.

I hope you find a way to do your Downward Dog without creating pain. If you feel a stretch sensation in your back, shoulders, buttocks, hamstrings and/or calves when in this position, it is a clear message that you still have some work to do. As the final exercise in this progression, the Downward Dog is therefore part of your maintenance routine. By adopting the Alignment First Protocol and making it your daily movement practice, you will get better at this exercise.

3.B: Inner Thigh Stretch – supine wall assisted

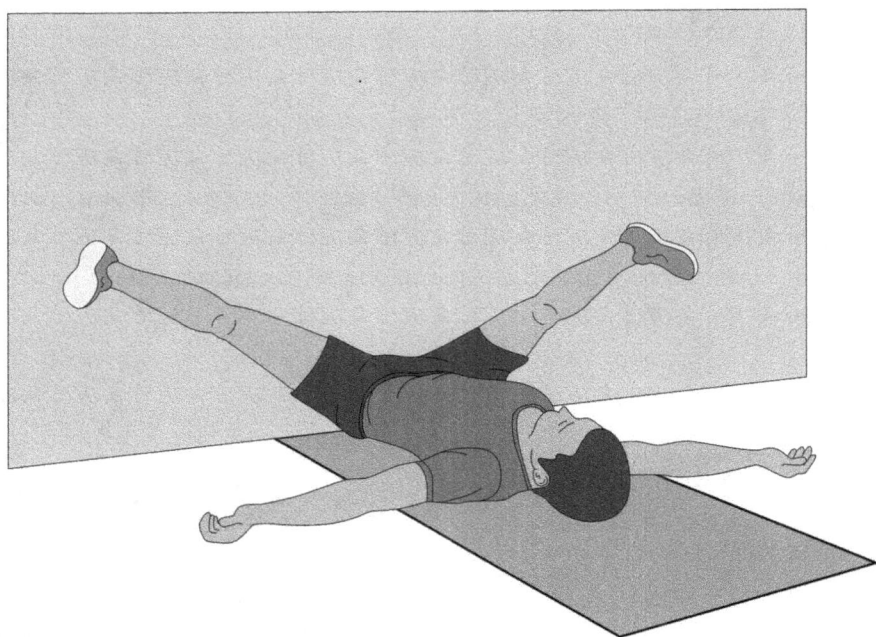

- Begin on your back with your legs up the wall and your body as close to the wall as possible, keeping your knees completely extended (unbent).
- Tighten your core muscles and begin practicing your deep breathing exercise.
- Keeping your knees fully extended and your toes pulled towards you (ankles dorsiflexed), move your feet as far apart as you comfortably can. Remain in that position for one minute.

Modifications

If this exercise caused or increased your pain, try the following modifications, as per the following sequence, until you can perform the exercise for one minute:

- If a rolled-up hand towel or a pool noodle helped with earlier on-your-back exercises, you will probably benefit from doing so in this exercise as well.
- Make sure you are tightening your core muscles as much as you are able.
- Limit how far your legs move apart during the exercise to lessen the tension in your inner thigh muscles and to potentially lessen the pressure in your hip joints.

If you can already separate your legs 90 degrees (normal hip abduction is considered to be 45 degrees per side), congratulations! It is now time to add a little more demand by graduating to the next exercise in this progression.

3.C: Groiner

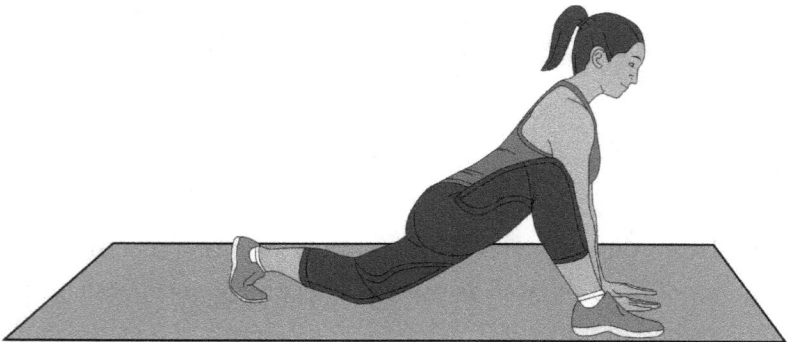

- Start on your hands and knees, with your arms and thighs as perpendicular to the floor as possible. Your hands should be shoulder-width apart and your knees should be hip-width apart. You your fingers should point straight ahead of you.

- Shift your weight onto your left knee and hand and bring your right foot out and around to rest on the floor, just outside of your right hand.
- With the toes of your left foot tucked under, slide your left foot and knee away from you along the floor. Keep your knee on the floor throughout the stretch.
- Tighten your core muscles as you try to lift your lower back and abdomen up away from the floor.
- Gently press your right knee out to the right, as far as you can, without losing the neutral position of your right foot.
- Settle into the stretch and maintain it for one minute. Repeat on the other side.

Modifications

If this exercise caused or increased your pain, try the following modifications, in the following sequence, until you can perform the exercise for one minute:

- Make sure you are tightening your core muscles as much as you are able.
- You can reduce how far you slide your rear leg back to lessen the tension in your inner thigh muscles and potentially, lessen the pressure in your hip joints.
- If you can't find a way to modify this exercise so it's comfortable for you, you may have to return to the previous version of the inner thigh stretch (3.B, supine wall assisted). Continue practicing it until your body is ready for the stability demanded by the Groiner. Test it weekly until your body gives you the green light to move ahead.

If you can already do the Groiner with little stretch sensation and with no pain or no increased pain, you're doing well. Move on to the next exercise in the progression, 3.D.

3.D: Inner Thigh Stretch – seated

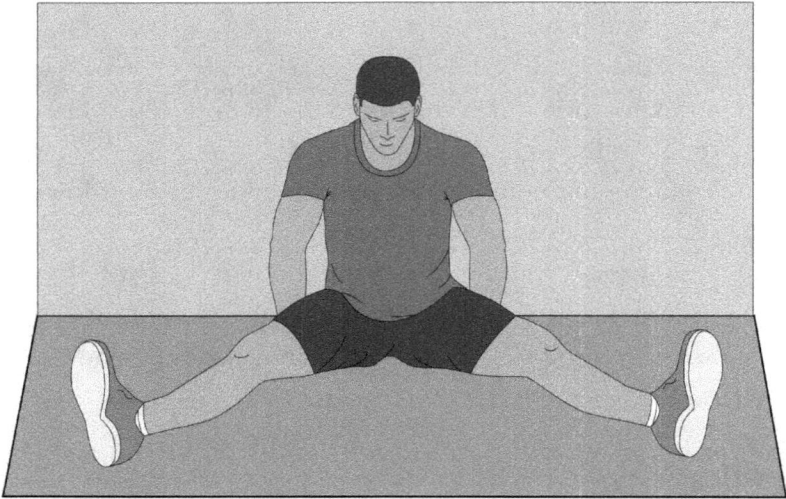

- Sit with your back against a wall and your legs out in front of you.
- Pull your toes towards you and straighten your knees as much as you're able.
- Tighten your core muscles, pushing your lower back into the wall as firmly as possible, while you separate your legs are far as they will comfortably go. If your upper back isn't flexed excessively, you should be able to hold your upper back and the back of your head against the wall without interfering with your ability to push your lower back into the wall.
- Take big, slow breaths and spend a minute in this position.

Modifications
- If you found this exercise to be pain-producing or pain-increasing, lessen how hard you are pulling your legs apart. This will probably do the trick.
- If pushing your lower back into the wall doesn't make any obvious difference to your comfort or performance in this stretch, try leaning forward to accentuate your stretch.

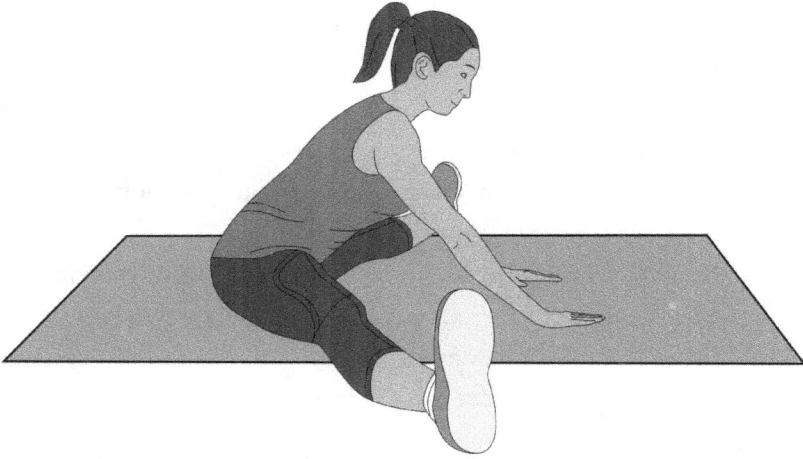

- When you can keep your spine straight and rigid while leaning forward to maximize your inner thigh stretch, you have achieved the gold standard of inner thigh stretching. This is also the inner thigh stretch that you will continue to do as part of your Alignment First maintenance routine.

4.B: Hip Flexor Stretch – kneeling

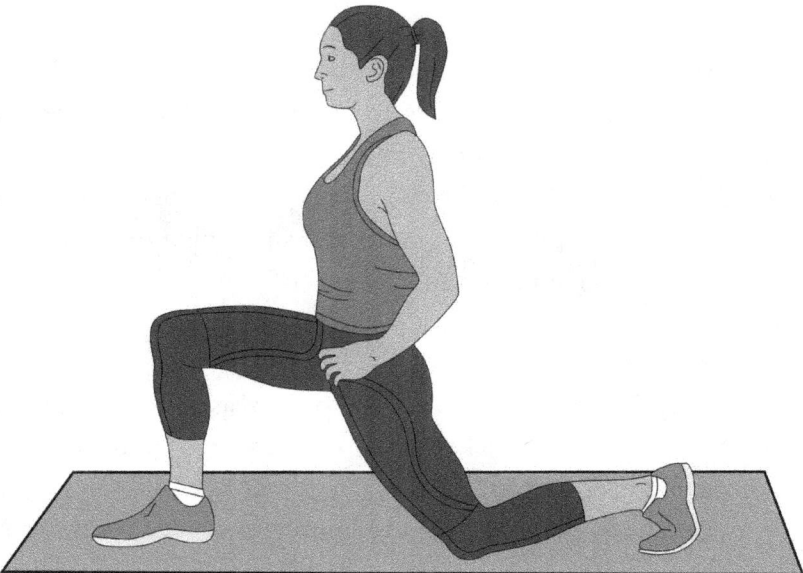

- Lower yourself down onto your left knee beside a large piece of furniture or a wall. This will give you balance/stability if you need it, as well as providing something you can brace yourself on, if you need help getting back up.
- To minimize any pressure discomfort in your left knee, kneel on a pillow, exercise mat or carpet.
- Place your right foot out in front of you so that your right knee and hip are both flexed to approximately 90 degrees.
- Tuck the toes of your left foot under and actively pull them towards your left knee (ankle dorsiflexed).
- Tighten your core muscles as much as you can and hold that tightness for the full minute of the stretch.
- Gently lunge forward far enough to create a stretch sensation in the front of your left hip and thigh.
- Try to keep your spine as vertical and rigid as possible. Try to lift your head towards the ceiling.
- Once you've pushed your pelvis as far forward as the lunge position allows, slide your right foot forward, in order to reacquire 90 degrees of knee flexion.
- Hold for one minute. Then switch sides and repeat.

I don't see many people who are chronically hip flexed. But I do see many who have their pelvis rotated too far forward. This exercise (and the Couch Stretch variations that follow) can be a powerful force for normalizing excessive forward rotation of the pelvis. Shortening of the hip flexor muscles, especially asymmetrical shortening of the iliopsoas muscle, is one of the most common causes of chronic lower back pain.

Modifications

- If you find this exercise causing or increasing lower back pain, try using less force. That should enable you to continue working on this exercise.
- Also, make sure you are maximizing your active core muscle tightening to protect the position and stability of your lower back.

- As you might imagine, knee pain is more common than back pain during this exercise. If your knees bother you, make sure you have plenty of padding between your knee and the floor. If your knee pain prevents you from doing this exercise, the alternative is the Side Lying Hip Flexor Stretch (see the following illustration). I'm not a big fan of this exercise because so many people have trouble stabilizing their lumbar spine in the side-lying position. Nevertheless, hypersensitive knees deserve to be accommodated.

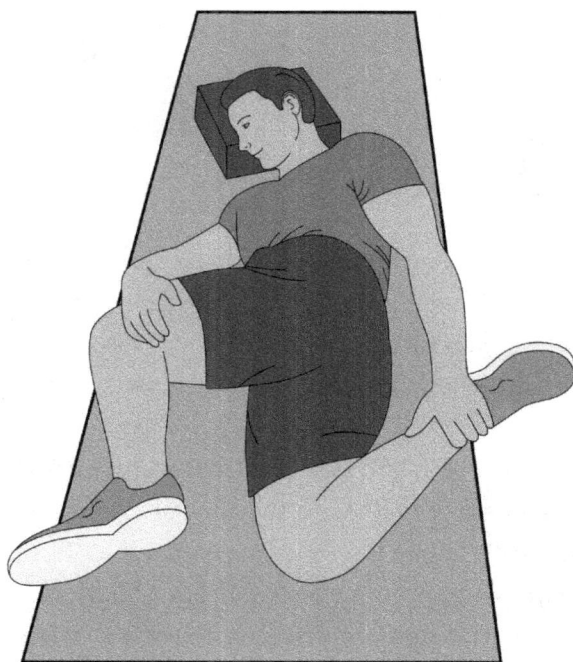

- If, on the other hand, you have no pain and can get full range of motion in hip extension (40 degrees) during the Kneeling Hip Flexor Stretch, you have earned the right to graduate to the next exercise in this progression. (4.C, Couch Stretch)

4.C: Couch Stretch – Position 2

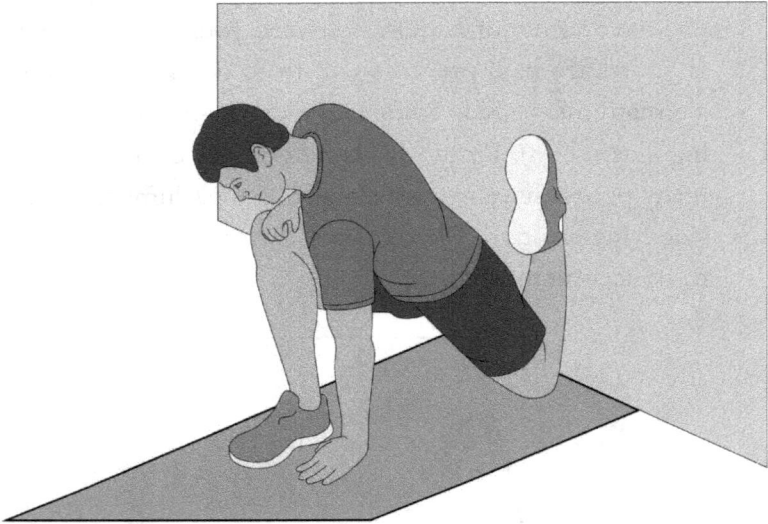

- Start this exercise on your hands and knees.
- To minimize the pressure discomfort in your knees, kneel on a pillow, exercise mat or carpet.
- Back up towards the wall, so that the soles of both feet touch the wall.
- Reach back with your left knee and place it in on your padding and against the wall, with your lower leg (shin/calf) and foot as vertically aligned on the wall as possible (Position 1).
- Shift your weight onto your left knee and hand, allowing you to bring your right foot out and around, to rest beside your right hand.
- Try to point your right foot directly ahead and gently pull your right knee to the right as far as you can without losing the neutral position of the foot.
- Tighten your glute and core muscles as much as possible and hold that tightness for the full minute of the stretch.
- Note. Although the picture of this exercise shows the person with one hand on his thigh, the majority of lower back pain patients

I work with, spend months getting good at this exercise with both hands still firmly on the floor.

- Repeat the stretch on the opposite side.

Modifications

Though this can be an aggressive stretch for some people, I've found that it rarely triggers lower back pain. The most common issue requiring a modification, is the stretch tension caused by having one foot all the way forward, beside your hand (Position 2). If this is your situation, fear not. It is perfectly legal to position your foot short of your hand in the beginning.

Try bringing your foot halfway to your hand (Call it Position 1.5), or even one quarter of the way (Position 1.25). Find a position for your foot that allows you to get a stretch into your hip/thigh, but not so much that it feels dangerous. Chip away at this challenge and before you know it, your hand and foot will be next door neighbors! Although this stretch appears to be very aggressive, I regularly have patients doing this exercise in my office and note this well: most of them have had knee surgeries, hip surgeries and even joint replacements! So. Put enough padding under the knee when necessary. Don't be overly aggressive. And find "your way" of making this extremely valuable exercise work for you.

4.D: Couch Stretch – Position 3

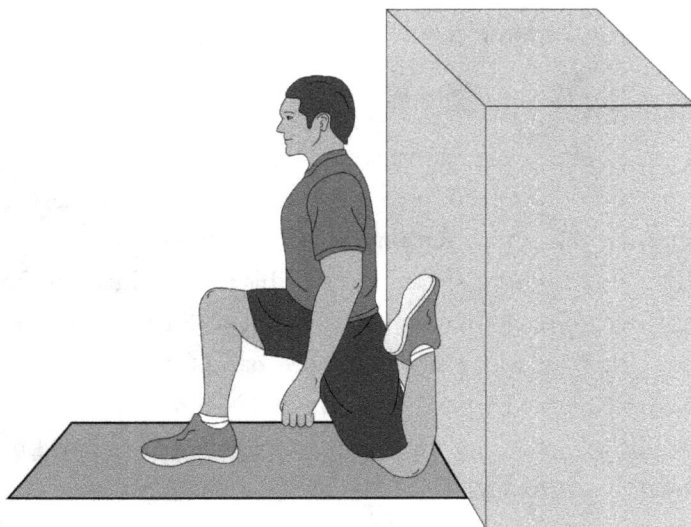

- Once you can comfortably perform the Couch Stretch in Position 2 (the previous exercise) for one minute you are ready to try Position 3, above.
- The only difference between the two exercises is that in Position 3, you bring your torso into as vertical a posture as possible.
- It is critical that you strongly contract your core muscles (coordinate and tighten your lower back and abdominal muscles) during this exercise to protect your lower back. Otherwise, any extra range of motion you get will likely come from spinal hyperextension rather than from hip extension.
- Tightening your glute muscles also helps to maximize the lengthening you are going to get out of your hip flexors (via reciprocal inhibition).
- When you can keep your spine straight and vertical in this exercise, you have reached the pinnacle of hip flexor stretching as far as the protocol is concerned. This is the hip flexor stretch that you will continue doing, as part of your Alignment First maintenance routine. Congratulations on achieving this milestone!

BTW: most people, when they first set out on this "journey of stretches", don't expect to ever conquer this exercise. And yet, most do.

5.B: Femur Rotations – seated

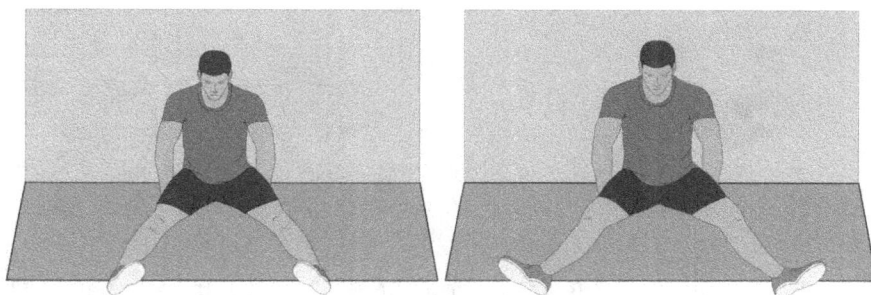

- The only difference between the Seated Femur Rotations and the Supine (on your back) version you've already done, is that this one is performed seated.
- Sit with your back and head against a wall, legs out in front of you and approximately three feet/one metre apart (the distance doesn't have to be exact).
- Pull your feet/toes towards you (ankles dorsiflexed) without bending your knees.
- Strongly pull your lower back into the wall by tightening your core muscles. Hold them like that for the duration of the exercise.
- While maintaining all the positional elements already mentioned, rotate your knees/feet towards one another and then away from one another, at a slow, steady pace, with just a slight pause at the end of each movement.
- Repeat 20 times.

This is a simple but important exercise progression. It helps you establish a neutral pelvic position and a stable lower back. This regular practice of rotating your hips will see you well prepared to keep your hip joints for a lifetime.

This exercise is also part of your maintenance routine, so over time you will get very good at it.

6.B: Hip Lift

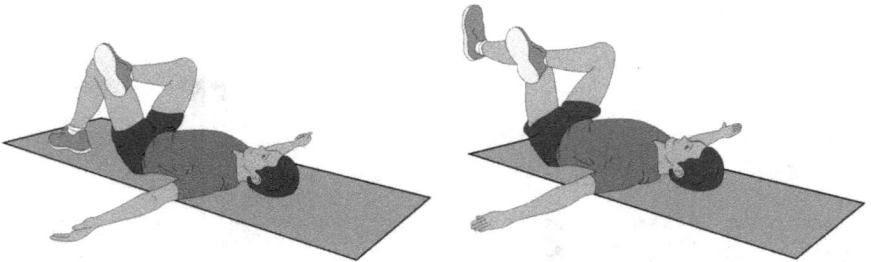

- Lie on your back with your knees bent to approximately 90 degrees and the soles of your feet flat on the floor.
- Place the outside of your right ankle on top of your left thigh just above your knee.
- Put your hands beside your body on the floor with palms down, to stabilize your upper body.
- Tighten your core muscles.
- Keeping your ankle "glued" in place on your thigh, lift your left knee towards your chest as far as is comfortable.
- The goal is to get at least 90 degrees of hip flexion and maintain that position for one minute.
- Repeat the exercise on the other side for one minute as well.

This exercise is all about producing a strong contraction in your hip flexor muscles. As always, be alert for imbalances between the two sides of your body in terms of mobility, "tightness" and discomfort. If you find that you are significantly less mobile on one side, you might want to double up your efforts on that side (i.e. activate left, then right and finally, the left side once more). By doubling the number of stretches on the less mobile side, you should be bringing your body into balance.

Modifications

- If you've been using a roll/noodle under your lower back in other exercises that have you on your back, you had better also try it here.
- If, when attempting this exercise, you feel pain, in either your lower back or your hip, you will have to return to the Modified Dead Bug (6.A, Chapter 9), for the time being. Retest the Hip Lift once a week, until you can do it without creating pain or increased pain

If you can produce at least 90 degrees of hip flexion and maintain the position for a minute, on both sides of your body, it is time for you to move on to the next exercise in this progression.

6.C: Lower Body Russian Twist x 10

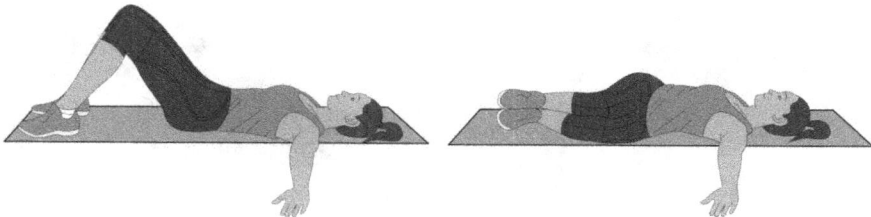

- Lie on your back with your knees bent to approximately 90 degrees and the soles of your feet flat on the floor.
- Put your hands at shoulder height on the floor with palms down, to stabilize your upper body.
- There are three distinct levels to this exercise. Keep your core muscles tight and your feet/knees together during each version of the exercise.
- At first, you will keep your feet on the floor and your knees together, as you gently lower your knees towards the floor on one side, and then the other.
- The next level is to take your feet off the floor, with knees bent, and trying to maintain 90 degrees of hip flexion (knees directly

over your hips) (and knees together), as you gently lower your knees first to one side of your body, and then to the other side.

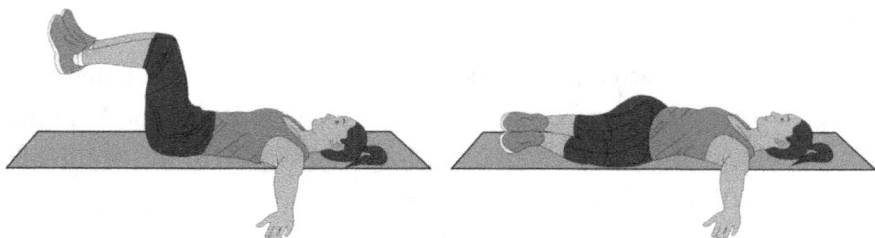

- The last version is to do the exercise with your knees completely straight, or very nearly so.

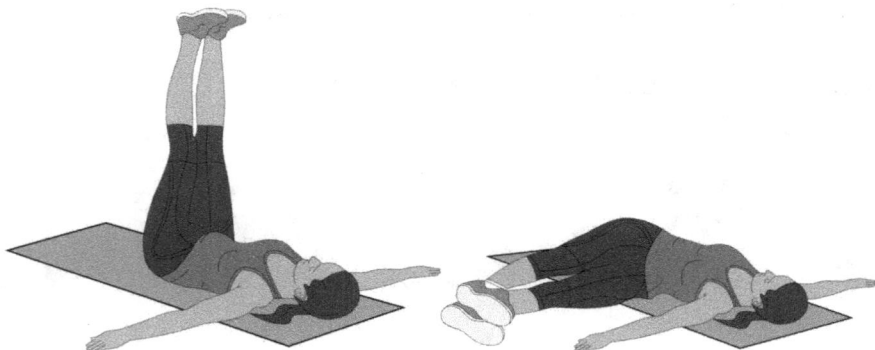

- Keeping your upper body in place, hold your knees together as you gently lower your knees first to one side of your body, and then to the other side.
- In this exercise, you only count the reps as you make the rotation back to the starting position. Don't credit yourself with ten repetitions when you have only completed five.

As you make progress in this exercise, you are strengthening every core muscle you own. Over the years, I've had a few chronic, lower back pain patients tell me that they believed this exercise, above all others, made the biggest difference to their lives.

Modifications

- If when attempting this exercise, you feel pain, return either to the Hip Lift or the previous version of the Russian Twist, that was pain-free. Retest the exercise that is interfering with your progress once a week, until you can do it without creating pain or increased pain

If you can perform 10 controlled repetitions of this exercise with straight legs, with at least 90 degrees of hip flexion and with no increased pain, it is time for you to graduate to the last exercise in this progression.

6.D: Straight Spine Sit Ups x 20

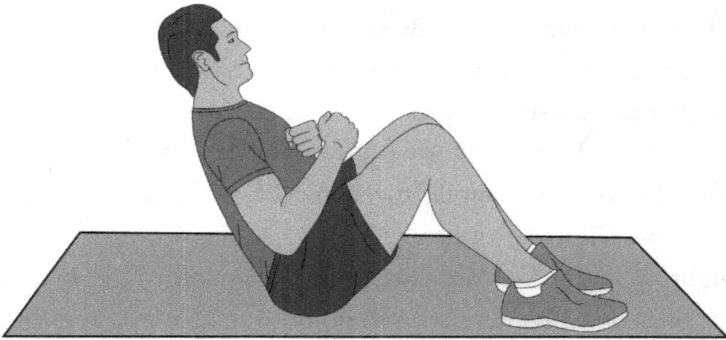

- Sit (as shown) on your back with your feet and knees hip-width apart, and your knees bent to approximately 90 degrees; then secure your feet under an immovable object.
- Tighten your core muscles strongly and cross your arms over your ribcage, tucking your hands under your arms. This will add stability to your torso.
- Keeping your spine as straight and as rigid as possible, slowly lower the back of your head towards the floor. Gently touch the back of your head to the floor and then lift your upper body, returning to the starting position. Touch only the back of your head to the floor. Do not touch or rest, any other part of your body to the floor.

- Your goal is to eventually complete twenty repetitions.

This is the toughest exercise in this exercise progression, but as long as you can stabilize your core, all the flexion occurs at your hips, protecting your lower back.

Modifications:

- If when attempting this exercise, you feel pain, return to the Lower Body Russian Twist. Then retest this sit-up exercise once a week, until you can do it without creating pain or increased pain

If you can perform 20 controlled repetitions of this exercise with a straight spine, through a healthy range of motion, you likely haven't had lower back pain for a while. By the time you do achieve this level of function, the Alignment First Protocol will have helped you improve bony alignment, muscle balance and stability. If you're at this point (or, when you do get here), the good news is that you will be an unlikely candidate for run-of-the-mill, mechanically-induced lower back pain. The bad news? There is none.

Straight Spine Sit Ups are part of the Alignment First maintenance routine, but I actually prefer you to do both the Sit Ups and the Lower Body Russian Twist. Or at least alternate them (daily or weekly). If you can perform these exercises properly, the combination of the two will provide a variety of core stimulation that is incredibly healthy, particularly for someone with a history of chronic lower back pain.

7.B: Cats and Dogs x 20

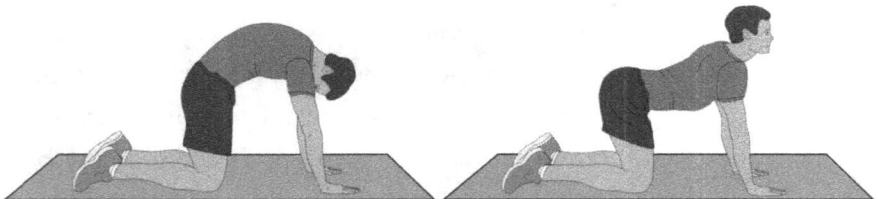

- Go on your hands and knees, with your arms and your thighs as perpendicular to the floor as possible.
- The goal of this exercise is to flex your entire spine and extend it through as large a range of motion as possible, without losing the good vertical position of your arms and thighs.
- A couple things will help you achieve proper technique in this exercise. First off, initiate the Cat part of the exercise by tucking your tailbone and chin towards one another. Doing so will help you forcefully exhale during this movement.
- Then, when you are ready to extend into the Dog part of the exercise, try to lift the tailbone and the top of your head toward the ceiling. It will also help if you inhale a large breath, as you move into this position.
- You don't need to pause in either of these positions for more than a second. In this exercise, the magic is in the movement.

Modifications

If you found this exercise to be pain-producing or pain-increasing, simply try moving through a smaller range of motion. Avoid the painful range and continue on. As you practice this routine, your body should gradually give you permission to move further in this exercise.

If, in spite of your best efforts, this continues to be painful, it will be better to return to Child's Pose (7.A in Chapter 9) until your body tells you it is ready for Cats and Dogs. Retest this exercise once a week, until your body gives you the green light to start practicing Cats and Dogs.

If you can do 20 full-range movements in this exercise, you need to start practicing Floor Twist.

7.C: Floor Twist

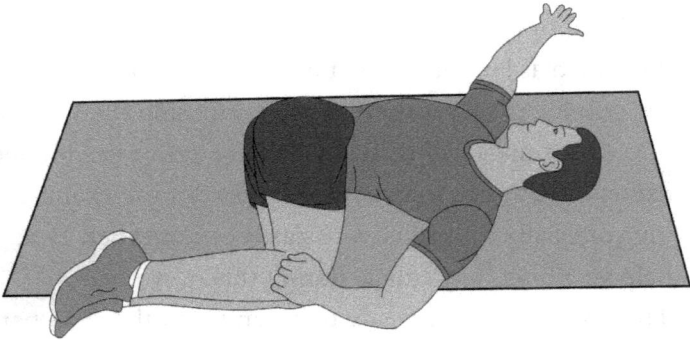

- Lie on your left side, with your hips and knees flexed to approximately 90 degrees.
- You may need a pillow for your head, to support your neck is a comfortable position.
- Tighten your core muscles to stabilize your lower back.
- Place your left hand on the front of your knees. This helps you to keep track of the vertical alignment of your knees. If you keep your knees stacked like that, it will help you to get the most out of this exercise. If you lose that ideal positioning, this exercise turns into a run-of-the-mill shoulder stretch.
- Place your right hand on the outside of your right knee, and keeping your elbow straight, lift your right hand up and over your torso diagonally. I want your hand to end up behind you, and also slightly overhead. Ideally your right arm should be approximately 45 degrees to your torso.
- As long as you have no acute neck problems, slowly, gently turn your head to look at your right hand.
- Practice your deep breathing exercise and let gravity do its thing.
- Allowing the arm to drop more directly behind you, lessens the stretch in your torso; and lifting the arm too close to your head is often uncomfortable, in either the shoulder or the neck.
- After one minute in this position, turn over and repeat the stretch on the other side.

Modifications

- It is quite rare for this exercise to trigger pain in someone with lower back pain. If you find it painful, try restricting your range of motion with a pillow, foam roll or something similar.
- If you are unable to find a way to do this exercise comfortably, then set it aside for the time being and return to Cats and Dogs. Retest Floor Test weekly, until it no longer causes pain.

If you experienced no trouble or discomfort during this exercise, move on to the next exercise.

7.D: QL Stretch

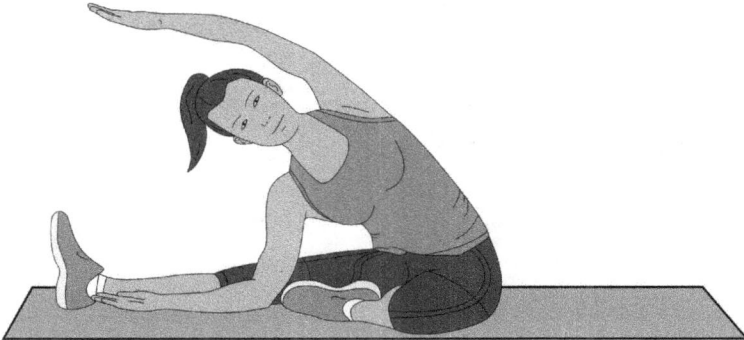

- Sit on the floor with your legs straight and as far apart as is comfortable.
- Push your knees into the floor to keep them straight and pull your toes towards your knees. Try to make your kneecaps and feet point directly up.
- Bend your left knee so that the sole of your left foot comes to rest against the inside of your right thigh.
- Drop your right forearm to the floor just to the inside of your right knee.
- Keeping your nose pointed straight ahead, side-bend your body to the right as if you are trying to put your right ear on your right knee.

- Reach your left hand directly overhead towards your right foot.
- Breathe deeply and slowly in that position for one minute.
- Repeat going to the left.

This is another one of those exercises where there aren't really any good modifications that don't completely change the nature of the exercise. If this exercise causes pain and simply doing it "less hard" doesn't eliminate the pain, return to the Floor Twist for a while. Retest QL weekly until it isn't pain producing.

This exercise is part of the Alignment First maintenance routine. It can be a very challenging exercise for some, but the rest of the protocol is designed to help you make progress with this exercise, as well as the others. Chip away at the process and you will improve your performance. I know, it sounds like work and I guess it is. But hey, every advancement to a new exercise is a step closer to relieving your pain problem.

8.B: Calf Stretch – standing

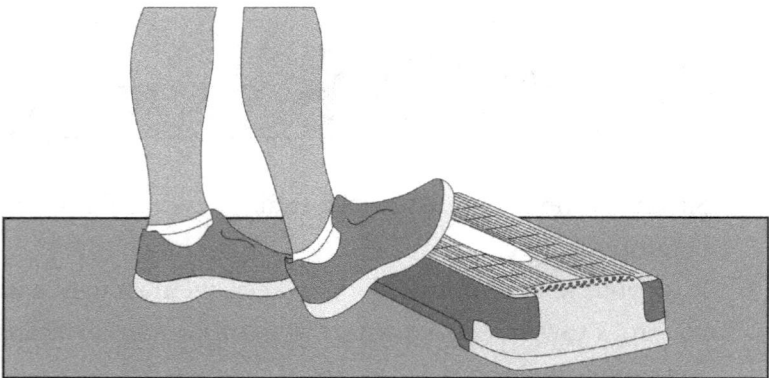

- You need to find an object to use to elevate the ball of your foot, up off the floor. The options of what to use are endless. Some people use a specially made slant board, a piece of wood or a half foam roll. If your ankle dorsiflexion range of motion is quite restricted (normal is considered to be 20 degrees), something that is a couple inches thick should be sufficient.

- Hang onto something with one or both hands for balance.
- Begin by placing as much of your weight as possible on the heel of your right foot.
- Lift the ball of your right foot as far off the ground as possible and move your block of wood under the ball of your foot (ideally touching or almost touching).
- With your knee as straight as possible, push your right hip forward until you feel a comfortable amount of stretch sensation in your right calf and/or foot.
- Hold for one minute and then, repeat on the left side.

Modifications

- If you found this exercise to be pain-producing or pain-increasing, you need to try using less pressure in the stretch.
- A smaller object under the ball of your foot may also help.
- Try bending your knee slightly.
- If these suggestions do not lessen or eliminate the pain produced by the exercise, you may have to return to the Supine Calf Stretch (8.A, in Chapter 9) for the time being. Retest the Standing Calf Stretch exercise once a week, until the pain is no longer being produced.
- If you happen to have significantly greater range of motion than 20 degrees of ankle dorsiflexion (say, 40 degrees or more), you need to be doing Calf Raises (8.C, below) rather than Calf Stretches. When it comes to feet and ankles, there is definitely such a thing as too much range of motion. If this is you, it is very important to do everything you can to develop enough strength and stability to control all that mobility you have.
- If you do not experience any aggravated symptoms when you do this exercise, try using a wall as your obstacle.

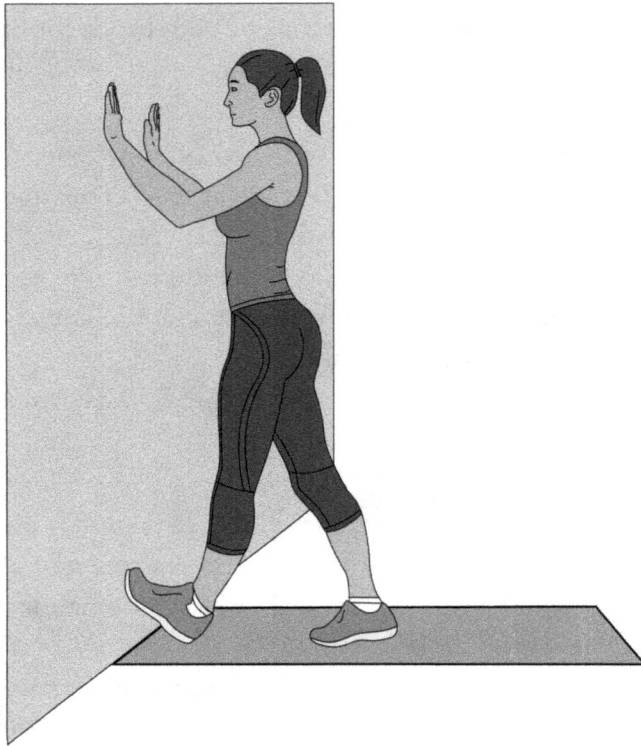

- It can be awkward for some people to use a wall for this exercise. And simply impossible if you don't already have sufficient mobility. If you can make it work for you, however, it is a convenient tool to use. And whether you end up using a wall or another tool, this exercise is part of the Alignment First maintenance routine. Keep your feet and calves stretched out and you should enjoy them for the rest of your life.

8.C: Stairway Calf Raises

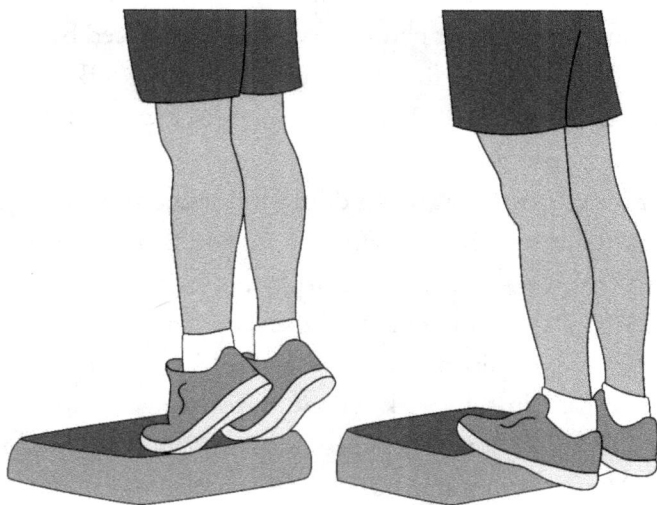

- Stand on a stair in your stairway, with your feet parallel and the balls of your feet supported on the edge of the stair. Keep your heels suspended in mid-air.
- Use a wall or banister, or both, for balance.
- Keeping your knees fully extended, rise up onto the balls of your feet as high as possible. Pause there a second before slowly lowering your heels as far as you can.
- Repeat 20 times.

Note: As I said earlier, if you have significantly greater range of motion than 20 degrees of ankle dorsiflexion (say, 40 degrees or more), these Calf Raises can help you develop the strength and stability you need to control all that mobility. Remember: when it comes to feet and ankles, there is definitely such a thing as too much range of motion.

Modifications

It is uncommon for someone to have pain with bodyweight Calf Raises and yet be able to do the Standing Calf Stretch without pain. Nevertheless, if you find the raises to be pain-producing or pain-increasing, try bending your knees slightly and try using a slightly smaller range of motion.

If this does not lessen or eliminate the pain produced by the exercise, you may have to return to the Standing Calf Stretch (8.B above), for the time being. Retest the Calf Raise exercise once a week, until the pain is no longer being produced.

It is very important that when doing this exercise, you do your best to maximize your range of motion without compromising good biomechanics. In this way, you can optimize the functional abilities of your feet and ankles for the long haul. Those of us in the rehab, fitness and therapy sector, are realizing that foot and ankle function plays a much more pivotal role, in things like squat performance, than we ever suspected (I credit Donnie Thompson for drawing this matter to my attention). When you master this exercise, your feet will thank you.

9.B: Bird Dog

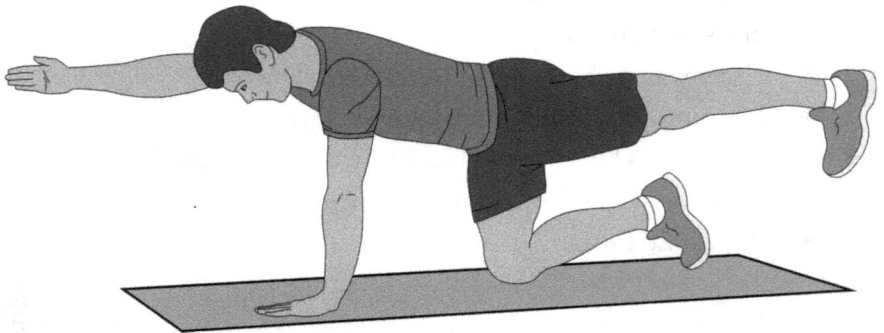

- This exercise begins with you on your hands and knees, with your arms and your thighs perpendicular to the floor.
- The object of this exercise is to get your entire spine as parallel to the floor as possible. Then lift one arm (i.e. right arm) and opposite thigh (i.e. left thigh) so that they, too, are as parallel to the floor as possible, without losing the good neutral position of your spine.

- Although the goal is to hold this position for 30 seconds on each side, you may have to break that 30 seconds into smaller chunks. It is not unusual, in fact, for lower back pain patients to begin with chunks of ten seconds or less.
- I have also found that for anyone with chronic lower back pain, the knee lift and hip extension can be difficult, at first. Many people tend to lose control of their pelvis/spine, on one side or both. If this seems to be happening to you, I recommend you keep your foot on the ground. It will add stability and control on your hip extension side.

Modifications

If you found this exercise to be pain-producing or pain-increasing, please experiment with the following modifications, in the order given, until you can perform the exercise for 30 seconds on each side:

- Do your best to tighten your core muscles strongly, in order to hold your torso rigid and protect your lower back.
- Make sure the foot on the extending hip side is still on the floor to add stability. Only begin lifting that foot up off the floor (on the hip extension side) when you are pain-free in your lower back.
- Trying to lift your arm "too high" will often create an extension in the lower back. Don't try to lift your arm higher than what your body can manage. Use your ability to maintain stability and a proper position of your spine, as your guide.
- Remember we are trying to keep the entire spine parallel with the floor, so don't lift your head. Keep your nose pointed at the floor.

When you can perform this exercise without trouble or discomfort, move on to the next exercise (9.C) in this progression.

9.C: Forearm Plank

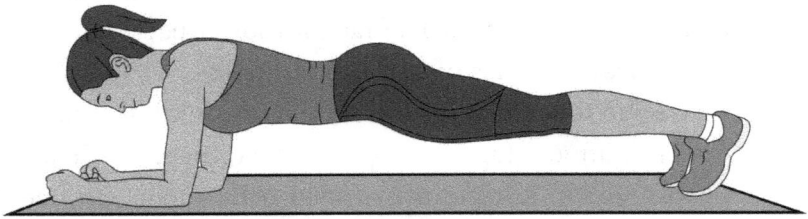

- From your hands and knees, lower yourself down onto your forearms and toes, with your entire body as straight and stiff as possible. Do not allow either your lower back or your hips to sag toward the floor.
- Although the goal is to hold this position for one minute, you may initially have to break that up into smaller chunks of time. It is not unusual, for lower back pain patients to begin by accumulating ten second efforts (i.e. hold the pose for 10 seconds, and then repeating it 6 times).

Modifications

- If you found this exercise to be pain-producing or pain-increasing, you need to make sure you are doing everything you can to tighten your core muscles.
- If you continue to struggle with this exercise, you can revert to a kneeling version. Retest the "full body" version weekly, to determine when you're ready to add this version to your routine.

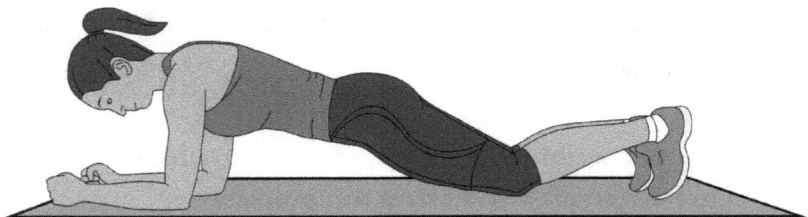

If you experienced no trouble or discomfort during this exercise, move on to the Side Plank version of the exercise.

9.D: Forearm Side Plank

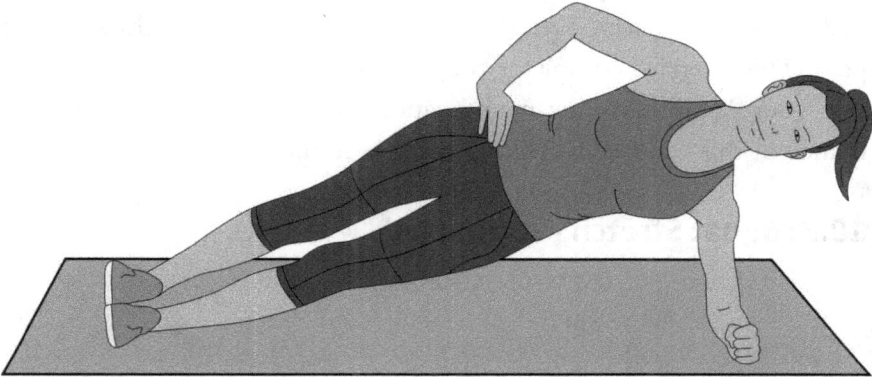

- From the floor, get up onto your left forearm and the outside of your left foot.
- Stack your right foot on top of your left foot and keep your nose pointing straight ahead.
- Keep your entire body as straight and stiff as possible. Tighten your core muscles as hard as you can. Do not allow your right hip to sag toward the floor.
- Although the goal is to hold this position for one minute, you may initially have to break that up into smaller chunks of time. It is not unusual, for lower back pain patients to begin by accumulating ten second efforts (i.e. hold the pose for 10 seconds, and then repeating it 6 times).
- Redo this exercise on your right side.

Modifications

- If you found this exercise to be pain-producing or pain-increasing, you need to make sure you are doing everything you can to tighten your core muscles.
- If you continue to struggle with this exercise, you can revert to a kneeling version. Retest the "full body" version weekly, to determine when you are ready to make that version part of your routine.

If you experienced no trouble or discomfort during this exercise, that is a significant accomplishment. People who have good bony alignment and a strong Forearm Side Plank do not generally have chronic back pain. This exercise completes progression 9 and is to be carried over into your Alignment First maintenance routine. As such, your performance of this exercise will likely improve immensely.

10.B: Squat Stretch - supported

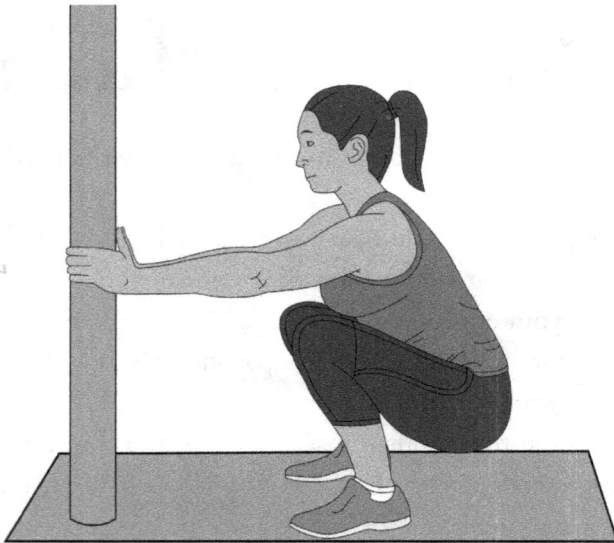

- Perform this exercise on a floor that is not slippery or wear footwear that will provide slip protection.
- Find an immovable object you can hold onto. I have patients do this in a doorway, holding onto the door frame.
- Place your feet approximately hip width apart (6-8") and squat down as low as possible, flaring your knees as wide apart as possible ("like a frog").
- Tighten your core muscles strongly, as you try to firmly pull your hips as far forward as possible.
- If you're like most people, in the beginning you will have to concentrate on pulling your knees as wide apart as possible, while

continually adjusting your feet back to parallel. Your ability to create this difference in positioning (dissociation) between your feet and knees is key to this exercise. It will be incredibly beneficial to them both.

- Practice your deep breathing exercise while you maintain this position for one minute.
- There is no modification for this exercise. This exercise is, in effect, a modification itself. If pain prevents you from doing it, you should return to the Supine Wall Squat Stretch (10.A, in Chapter 9). Retest this squat stretch weekly, to determine when you are ready to make it part of your routine.

If you had no discomfort problems with this exercise, please graduate to the next exercise in this progression.

10.C: Wallsit

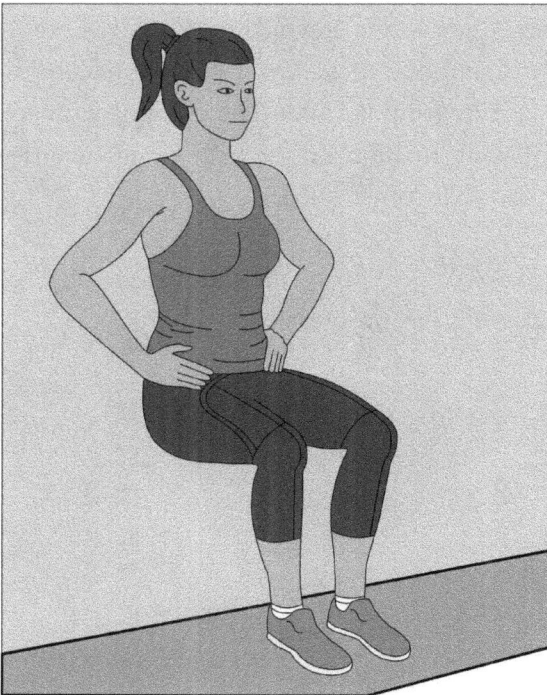

- Do this exercise on a floor that is not slippery, or wear footwear that will provide you with some slip protection.
- Back up to the wall and press your back and the back of your head against it. Position your feet and knees approximately hip width apart (6-8").
- Slide your body down the wall, until your hips and knees are bent to approximately 90 degrees.
- Tighten your core muscles firmly. Push your lower back into the wall.
- Now that you are in this position, the final positional element is to pull your knees slightly further apart than your feet. This helps to improve your foot and ankle positioning.
- Practice your deep breathing exercise while you maintain this position on the wall for one minute.

Modifications

- The only real modification for this exercise is to not lower yourself quite so far down. If discomfort does force you to sit a little higher on the wall, you may have to adjust the distance your feet are from the wall. The object is to ensure that regardless of your position on the wall, your lower legs are vertical when viewed from the side.

If you had no discomfort problems with this exercise, please graduate to the last exercise in this progression.

10.D: Deep Squat

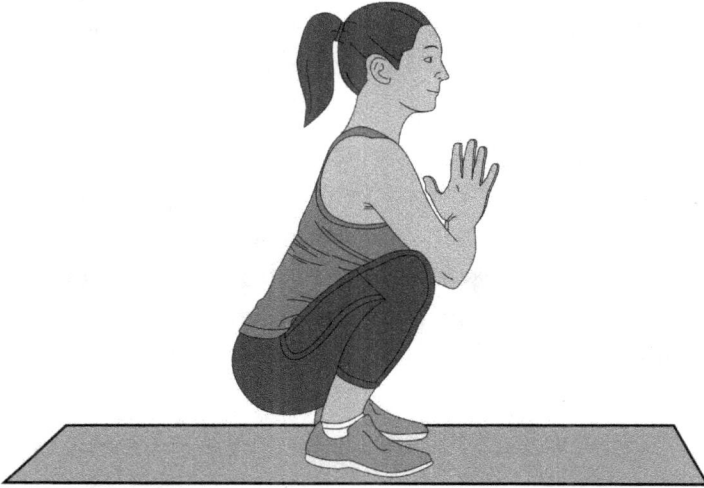

- Do this exercise on a floor that is not slippery, or wear footwear that will provide you with some slip protection.
- The Supported Squat Stretch has helped you develop the mobility you need to transition to a "look ma, no hands" squat. You no longer need to hold onto anything for support. That's the only difference between the two exercises.
- The Wallsit has provided you with the necessary strength to maintain a deep squat position without holding on for support.
- Place your feet approximately hip width apart (6-8") and squat down as low as possible, flaring your knees as wide apart as possible ("like a frog").
- Tighten your core muscles strongly, as you try to firmly pull your hips as far forward as possible.
- Now that you are no longer holding on for support, you should not have to continually adjust your feet back to parallel; but keep an eye on their positioning just the same.
- Practice your deep breathing exercise while you maintain this position for one minute.

Modifications

- The one common modification for this exercise is a need to place your feet slightly wider apart than 6-8 inches. That is fine so long as you keep your feet parallel to one another, and no further apart than your knees.
- If changing your foot placement doesn't help you enough, you have to decide between two options before proceeding. You can simply hang on for balance (thus returning to the Supported version of the exercise). Your other option is to return to the Wallsit but this time, allow your hips to drop below the level of your knees.

If you've had no discomfort problems with this exercise, congratulations: you've just graduated from Body Mechanic's School!

By working your way through this corrective exercise protocol, you have done what many people are unwilling to do. You've persevered and in so doing, regained control of your biomechanical health. It's been my experience, that those who perform the Alignment First Maintenance Routine escape the clutches of lower back pain.

How do you feel? I expect that the body you have today is more capable and certainly, more comfortable than the one you had before you purchased this book (and practiced the protocol).

Now let's move on and explore what happens next. Chapter 11 is for you whether you've had tremendous success, some success or surprisingly little.

CHAPTER 11

What Now?

*"Success is achieved and maintained by those
who try and keep trying."*
— W. Clement Stone

By now, I assume you have experimented with — and may even be practicing — some of the exercises of the Alignment First Protocol. I'm hoping that you've already enjoyed some success with these exercises or at least, you can feel their inherent promise. As I mentioned at the beginning of this book, the timespan for the process of improvement is unique to each of us.

Keep in mind that the protocol is full of healthy and safe demands designed to improve your body's alignment, function and comfort. And know that the author of this book (yes, that's me) wants you to get the utmost from your exercises. I appreciate how disappointing it is to have experienced pain relief only to discover it's only temporary. I expect you've experienced some of this frustration, along the way. I say let's leave the frustration behind and work the protocol.

I'm guessing your body took years to get into its misalignment, so it's going to take some time to get it back into alignment. Your job is to become proficient at each of the exercises on the list. Doing so won't get you a spot on the Olympic team, but it should keep you "in the game", whatever your game is. Homemaker, weekend warrior, desk jockey or all three: when you get the hang of these exercises, you will develop a degree of muscle balance and postural integrity that will set you apart from most of your peers.

Those proficient in these exercises do not typically have sore backs (or sore hips, knees or feet). Nor do they typically end up needing back surgery or joint replacements. Remember Nike's 'Just Do It' slogan?

For too many of us, it engendered an attitude that said, get "it" done, whatever "it" was, regardless of the cost. Much better, I think, to adopt an enlightened mantra, like: "Get straight. Move better. Feel great."

That mantra leads into the conundrum that all pain, physio and rehab specialists encounter, time and time again. Most patients agree that pain is the ultimate motivator. It is the human condition to avoid pain as much as possible and to seek relief from it. And yet, the number of people who stop doing their exercises – or treatments – the minute their pain subsides, is astounding. It is as if they forgot how uncomfortable their pain was.

I can understand long-term, chronic pain sufferers being unable to remember being pain-free. I get that. But what astounds me is how little time it takes some patients to forget what chronic pain feels like. Whether their memories are surprisingly short or amazingly selective, this lapse always baffles me.

People who completely embrace the lessons of the Alignment First Protocol will not require those lessons until the end of time. But if they think they can teach their body just enough to pass the test for the time being, they're wrong. If they relinquish their daily regimen, their bodies will gradually return to their original posture with its pain and awkwardness of movement.

I hope it doesn't happen to you but if it does, if you should experience a return to pain, you will have to start all over again. You need that sequential process to rebuild a healthy balance in your muscles and joints. If you can make these exercises part of your daily ritual, you'll be able to convert your back pain from an ever-present companion into a fading memory. That's an amazing payoff for not all that much work!

Now, let's talk about "what if you didn't enjoy much success with the exercises?". What if you worked hard on the Alignment First Protocol for two or three months and your lower back pain hasn't disappeared. What now? Here follows a way to assess your situation and move forward with some degree of confidence.

If you experienced less than 100% success with Alignment First, you fall into one of four categories:

1. Not There Yet
2. Persistent Malalignment
3. "The Little Kicks Syndrome"
4. Neurological Overwhelm

1. Not There Yet

If you are feeling better as a result of the Alignment First exercises, but are not yet pain-free, you are likely on the right path. Your body may just need more time. You're asking a lot of it. Postural reorganization. Soft tissue healing. Increased range of motion. Your body has been coping with, and compensating for, the imbalances responsible for your lower back pain for how long? Years? Decades? Healing takes time as does becoming accustomed to your new alignment. Chiropractors call this lag the "post-adjustment healing cycle".

In complex cases, the cycle can easily take over a year. If you have felt some improvement of symptoms, but not as much as hoped, you probably need more time. Time to get better at the exercises. Time for your body to properly reorganize, heal and learn healthier movement patterns. If you're feeling better but are not yet pain-free, you're not yet far enough down the path to feel great. Other than immediate, dramatic pain reduction, this time lag is the most common response to the protocol.

2. Persistent Malalignment

The next likeliest reason for a lack of immediate success with the Alignment First Protocol, is the presence of an alignment problem that the exercises are not correcting. There are some functional and structural reasons for such a situation.

In the healthcare world, we talk about the *primary lesion*. The root cause of the problem. My favourite analogy of this concept comes from Julien Pineau, a movement, strength and conditioning coach in southern California. As a boy, he saw a documentary about logging companies floating logs downriver. Whenever a log jam occurred (and they did), the companies would call out their resident engineering expert. He'd identify the one "key log" that, when removed, would untangle the jam and allow the flow of logs to resume.

Using this analogy, the key log is the primary lesion. Find it, eliminate it as the source of trouble and many other related troubles are often washed away in the process. Some "key lesions" can be corrected with the Alignment First Protocol. Some cannot.

Functional Reasons

There are some functional asymmetries that are not well addressed by the Alignment First Protocol. In my experience, the majority of people who do not experience success with these exercises have an alignment problem at C1 (the first bone in the spine, below the skull, is called *C1*). Misalignment of C1 can cause an incredible variety of symptoms that most people would never attribute to a problem in the neck.

Indeed, had someone told me that C1 could cause so many issues, twenty years ago, I'd have looked at them in disdain. I'd have said that no problem in the neck could cause pain or dysfunction elsewhere in the body. Of course, a "crooked" bone in the neck might cause a headache or some neck pain. But could it cause lower back pain, a numb hip or 'tennis elbow' symptoms? No way, I'd have said. And very wrong I'd have been. Here's why.

NUCCA (National Association of Upper Cervical Chiropractic) is a chiropractic specialty based on the concept that the first cervical verte-bra is a unique bony structure in the body. Misalignment of that bone can cause all kinds of strange and unwelcome symptoms elsewhere in the body. The brainstem actually descends into an opening in the center of C1. Since there is not an abundance of "extra" room there, when C1 becomes misaligned, it can cause mechanical pressure directly upon the brainstem. It's like you poked it with a stick. Since muscle tone for the entire body is regulated therein, poking it with a stick doesn't seem to be a good idea if you can avoid it.

My interest in NUCCA was sparked by one of my most trying cases in the late 90s. A young woman had been in two serious car accidents that left her struggling with unrelenting chronic pain. I'd been working with her, two or three times a week, for years, doing my best to keep her head above water as she transitioned from one pain crisis to another. Then her status took an unexpected turn for the better as a direct result of a NUCCA correction.

Based on a recommendation from another patient, this woman drove 4 hours each way to be assessed and treated by a NUCCA practitioner. After years of working with her, I was very familiar with her posture and muscle tone. I was amazed at how dramatically improved both were following this first adjustment.

My belief in NUCCA's efficacy has continued to strengthen, since that experience. I've worked quite closely with many NUCCA practitioners for years, now. And then, in November of 2014, I had my own NUCCA experience.

I was moving some household effects. I'd partially pulled a carpet roll off the trailer and stood up under it, to take the weight onto my left shoulder. That's when I felt a sharp pain in my shoulder that went straight up the left side of my neck and into my head, above my left ear. I knew right away that I had injured myself.

Over the next couple of days, I worked on exercises to straighten and relax my tight and sore body. But nothing was easing the pain in my head and neck. The pain was constant. And then, a couple days after the injury, I developed a patch of superficial numbness centered on the point of my right hip. X-rays showed that my C1 had been pulled sharply down to the left side and that the entire bone had slipped upward, on the right side of my skull.

Dr. Jordan Ausmus, a NUCCA chiropractor, made the correction to my C1 position and the pain in my head and neck disappeared immediately. The numbness in my hip started to lessen over the next few days, and disappeared entirely, three weeks later. Even with all of my experience, I was astonished that the mechanical pressure in my neck (that lasted 5 days before being corrected), could cause symptoms in my hip that would last for three weeks AFTER being corrected. There is no explanation in any textbook for what I had experienced.

If I'd had any lingering doubts about the importance and efficacy of NUCCA care, I no longer did.

I remember my first mentor, Paul St. John, telling me that the jaw will tend to mimic the position of the pelvis. I am not aware of any research that supports his assertion, but it is an idea that has stuck with me over the years. It has certainly been my observation that malalignment of the pelvis can interfere with the neck to be well aligned, and vice versa. So, it is not that big of a stretch to include the jaw in that thought process.

There's another interesting relationship within the body that should be more widely recognized. It has to do with the way our teeth bite together ("occlusion") and how this can be influenced by alignment problems lower down, in the body. You can prove this to yourself. Gently tap your teeth together as you move your head. If your head tilts left, the teeth on the left typically hit first. If your head tips right, the teeth on the right hit first. The same thing applies to when you tip your head forward or back.

I learned that little "bite" of knowledge and much more about the science of occlusion from Dr. Curtis Westersund. He's a dentist who specializes in helping people improve their bite. If your teeth do not contact each other evenly, it can create more harm than just the accelerated wear and tear of your teeth (which is bad enough!). A misaligned bite has the potential to also create painful problems in ligaments and muscles of the neck and jaw. And more.

Occlusion is a complicated interaction of nerves, muscles and structures. A simple opening and closing of your jaws is quite a feat of biomechanical precision. When there is a big alignment problem in the skeleton, your body does everything possible to provide perfect occlusion. But these muscular compensations fatigue the muscles that control the jaw (much as they do the muscles elsewhere in the body). Tired and sore jaw and neck muscles cause headaches, neck pain and/or jaw problems. And then, consistent with Pfluger's Laws, symptoms spread outward, potentially impacting the back and shoulders. Eventually, the entire body can become involved. In some instances, in spite of the best efforts to align and balance the body, faulty occlusion can get in the way.

Though there are some wonderful exceptions, most dentists are like the rest of the healthcare profession: unwilling or unable to acknowledge how their work is impacted by alterations in whole body alignment. But the evidence is clear. Just as patients with chronic, lower back pain can be helped by alignment and balance improvements in their hips and pelvis, they can also be helped by improvements as far away as in the neck, teeth and jaw.

Structural Reasons

Actual structural asymmetries are another explanation for little or no success with the Alignment First Protocol. Unfortunately, no amount of corrective exercise can remedy some disorders. These include having a condition called *hemipelvis*, characterized by having one side of your pelvis (ilium) be smaller than the other. Or you might have a structurally short leg, which can be genetic or due to injury. Or you might have a fallen arch or other structural differences between your feet. In fact, when people have had these kinds of left/right asymmetries for decades, it is typical for one foot (or both) to be collapsed to one degree or another.

If your feet do not create a strong, stable base of support, they can be the source of dysfunctional forces ascending throughout your body. The Alignment First Protocol can help you straighten your pelvis, hips and lower back, but if one or both of your feet are badly pronated, your improvements will likely be temporary. At least until the architectural problems in your foot/feet are addressed. Foot pronation tends to cause a predictable series of positional faults and compensations further up, in the skeleton. All of these alignment issues cause unnecessary stress and strain, typically resulting in irritation in the short term, and then transitioning to degenerative changes and chronic pain when persisting over the long term.

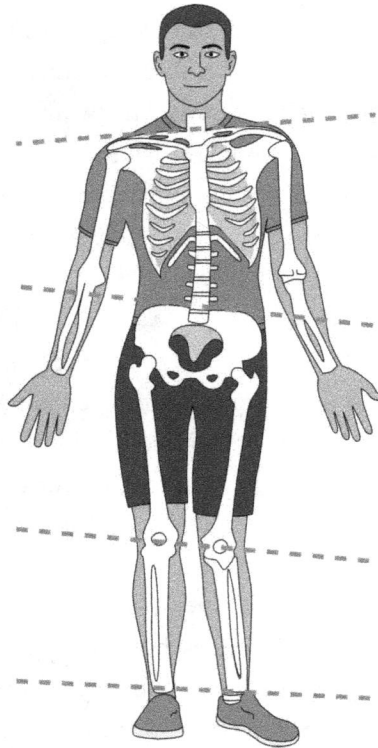

Wedge Posture

The Wedge Posture is a common and unstable way for the body to be organized. In an attempt to add stability, the body will often compensate by turning the feet out in an exaggerated manner to create a broader base of support. Others compensate by standing with their feet very far apart. The biggest problem with this particular compensation is that the more your feet turn outward, the less you are able to maintain neutral foot and ankle posture. When your feet point out like a duck, the soft tissue tension in your lower legs and feet, that normally help you maintain good arches, are prevented from doing so. If your feet are not pointing straight ahead, start now, today: practice keeping them as parallel as possible.

This parallel positioning of the feet can be so powerful that on occasion I see patients who actually regain normal foot posture with this single, simple modification. In fact, if you can't create reasonably neutral foot and ankle positioning by getting your feet parallel, when in one of the squat progression postures, you need to seek out professional help from a foot expert. Many functional asymmetries can be remedied with the Alignment First Protocol, but almost any structural asymmetry in the lower body will make it necessary for you to recreate symmetry through foot orthotics.

3. The Little Kicks Syndrome

What does "The Little Kicks Syndrome" refer to? In Season 8 of the television sitcom *Seinfeld*, Elaine showed off her dancing skills. It turned out that she had a comically disjointed way of dancing that she was completely unaware of. Many of us are similarly unaware that we hold or move our bodies in ways that are dysfunctional and even pain producing. These "habitual ways of being" are so deeply ingrained that no amount of mobilization and stretching will ever have any lasting impact. The nervous and muscular systems literally have to be retrained at a deeper level.

For these situations, there are two methodologies I have had varying degrees of success with. The first approach is called Somatic Re-education. This is an approach that was developed by Thomas Hanna. Hanna was a student of Moshe Feldenkrais, the creator of Functional Integration, which many people simply know as Feldenkrais.

The other approach is called Dynamic Neuromuscular Stabilization which was developed by Pavel Kolar, a Czech physiotherapist. Both of these systems are designed to re-educate the neuromuscular system. Whereas the Alignment First Protocol is primarily a "mechanical" method of postural reorganization, Somatics and DNS are neuromuscular approaches. There are practitioners who specialize in helping chronic pain sufferers with these systems.

My favourite book dealing with this type of training, and one of my all-time favorite books, is Thomas Hanna's *Somatics: Reawakening the Mind's Control of Movement, Flexibility and Health*. This book is an excellent resource for anyone wishing to supplement what they have learned in this book.

4. Neurological Overwhelm

Dr. John Sarno has written a number of books suggesting that the vast majority of chronic pain problems stem from something he calls *tension myoneural syndrome* (TMS). According to Dr. Sarno, pain is often created by the body as a way to divert attention away from troubling emotional issues. He believes that chronic pain patients can overcome this strategy to repress these powerful emotions by focusing their attention on the underlying emotional issues. The main point being that when the pain symptoms are seen for what they are, a distraction and nothing more, they will go away. This is an idea that is not currently accepted by the mainstream medical community.

While I am not a proponent of Dr. Sarno's work, I believe that the mind-body connection, at the very core of his message, is real and relevant to our discussion. The salient point of Dr. Sarno's theory is that the human nervous system has a finite capacity to cope with stimulation. This capacity is individual and elastic, but it is limited. (Remember the Smart Phone capacity metaphor from Chapter 2?)

Many factors impact how big and how full your "phone's storage" is, with both factors being subject to change. Any therapeutic intervention that decreases neurological input or that increases your capacity to cope with input will be helpful. Is it possible that successfully dealing with difficult emotional issues might also decrease neurological stress? I certainly think so. Is it possible that a positive expectation of such an outcome is reasonable and also, stress reducing? I believe it could be. That's why I am inclined to see Dr. Sarno's protocol for processing emotional upset as a potential tool to include in our pain-eliminating toolbox. We seldom need to use the more radical tools, but it is nice to know we have such options when things get complicated.

Another effective tool, to use when dealing with chronic pain, is respiration. I know 'breathing' sounds so simple but a review of the section on breathing, near the end of Chapter 6, is always a good idea. We humans have been avoiding and managing neurological overwhelm with yogic breathing and other similar approaches for thousands of years. And now, we are seeing a renaissance of yoga and yogic breathing for good reason. I encourage you to seek out a breathing practice that works for you and incorporate it into your daily routine. There are few things more health promoting. And given how life spans are getting longer, we might as well live those "extra" years on our feet rather than on our backs.

In this chapter, I've mused about what your experience with the Alignment First Protocol might have been (or might yet be). If you're feeling better already and experiencing less pain (a loss you're pleased to experience, I am sure), I'm glad for you. Some people respond to the protocol quite a bit faster than others. To you I say: please stick with your regimen. Your body will thank you, time and time again.

If you're feeling that the protocol has helped but not near as much as you'd hoped, I urge you to stick with it. Alignment and postural problems evolve over time; sometimes, over years. It may take a year or more to resolve those issues. Be patient. Exercise daily. And trust in the process. It has worked for thousands of people. It should work for you, too.

And for those of you who feel your search for lower back pain relief is still ongoing, know that I share your frustration. I've had patients tell me they're losing (or have already lost) interest in trying to navigate the healthcare universe. Too much information. And so much of it so contradictory. How do you know who to listen to?

By outlining some of the complications that might interfere with your search for comfort, I hope I've given you an insight on how you might direct yourself toward a future free from the clutches of debilitating lower back pain.

Conclusion

*"Perfection is not attainable,
but if we chase perfection we can catch excellence."*
— VINCE LOMBARDI

I wrote this book for two reasons: to provide a fundamental perspective on the mechanical causes of lower back pain and to offer a simple, step-by-step process for eliminating those causes.

You might say I took something Einstein said to heart: "If you can't explain something to a six-year-old, you don't understand it yourself". As you've read, we really do need to understand some things about our physiology before we can address chronic pain. You know it hurts and you know where that hurt is. But why does it hurt? What caused it? And how can we make it go away? To answer these questions, I felt it necessary to discuss a number of related issues.

I've explained concepts that may be well beyond the grasp of most six-year-olds. But I anticipate that you found the information more clarifying than confusing. I also hope you perceive what I very much want you to perceive: that the Alignment First Protocol and the principles it's built upon are disarmingly simple.

My other hope is, now that you've read this book, that you adopt these takeaways:

1. You're now armed with the knowledge you need to be your own Body Mechanic.
2. Pain is not a mysterious, luck-related affliction. There is a knowable cause of your lower back pain.
3. Although we are all skeletally unique, there is an ideal, three-dimensional bony alignment inside each of us. And we can train our bodies to approximate that postural model by using a

logical, step-by-step process of corrective exercise and supporting techniques.

4. The active pursuit of alignment excellence is the natural way to reorganize the body so it is no longer plagued with painful, inefficient postures.

5. When alignment is improved, comfort increases. Tissue health is enhanced. Mobility is restored. Strength and motor control problems are eased. Even mental outlook is often improved.

6. You must work intelligently and consistently on this process in order to maximize your long-term benefits. Imagine, benefits can include a future without the need for back braces, surgeries or pain medications.

7. If this system hasn't worked for you, there are specific healthcare professionals you need to seek out in order to assess your unique needs.

There are millions of people who struggle with chronic lower back pain. A huge percentage of them suffer as a direct result of misalignment of the skeleton, particularly the pelvis. And way, way too many of these people are giving up on trying to solve their pain problems because so many of their attempts have been frustratingly unsuccessful. These people need real help.

Chronic lower back pain patients are exposed to many misguided ideas, beliefs and treatments in regard to their pain problems. How can they solve a problem when they don't understand what's causing it? Or worse, how can they resolve an issue that they think they know the solution to, when they are in fact mistaken? I don't blame them for desperately surfing the web looking for answers, but I am aghast at much of the advice offered there. It's not only horribly wrong; some of it is downright dangerous.

If left uncorrected, chronic lower back pain problems can completely overwhelm people and dominate their lives. Sufferers don't have world class athletic aspirations. They're not asking for the moon. All they want is to get their lives back.

They need help understanding what's important and what's not important regarding their pain. They also need a logical, step-by-step process they can safely use to unwind the distorted postures that are causing their pain. What's needed, in most chronic lower back pain situations, is a perspective like that of the Alignment First Protocol.

Unfortunately, few healthcare practitioners focus on assessing or correcting malalignment in the body. I know, everyone just assumes chiropractors specialize in correcting alignment problems. Some do, NUCCA chiropractors being a notable example, but the majority specialize in restoring joint mobility. Their working assumption seems to be that improved mobility will naturally result in improved alignment. I am no fan of this assumption. Yes, it does help sometimes. But just as often, it doesn't help. To me, this issue is far too important to be left to chance.

At present, restoring mobility is the popular therapeutic path. But c'mon, people! How on earth can they expect their bodies to move skillfully through a full range of motion when they can't even organize their bodies into a neutral posture? I know. There are those of us who feel we're as fluid as Freddy Couples (PGA champ with lovely, long drives off the tee). But too often, we're more like Jim Furyk and his "unusual" golf swing (best described as "an octopus falling out of a tree"). While Jim's unorthodox biomechanics earn him millions of dollars in professional golf winnings, the rest of us are at risk of back surgeries and hip replacements.

So. Just because you can "get the job done" with wonky biomechanics doesn't mean it's a good idea. Don't let your pain deceive you. Its alarm may only sound in one part of your body – hips, back, neck or head – but remember, our bodies are more than just the sum of all of its parts. And they're all totally interconnected.

It is also not enough to dwell on one issue alone. It isn't "one" of the following: alignment, mobility, stability, motor control, strength or endurance. It is "all of them and all of them" in the order given. There is a logical and necessary order to the steps in the rehabilitation process, and respecting that order is necessary for predictable, successful outcomes.

Thousands of patients, from all walks of life, have proven the effectiveness of the Alignment First Protocol: from grandmothers and children to office workers and professional athletes. The principles upon which this system is built are solid, and when they are adhered to, there is success to be had along this path.

I trust the information I've shared with you has been helpful.

"If you can see things out of whack,
then you can see how things can be in whack."
— Dr. Seuss

Sincerely wishing you all the best in your search for a healthy and happy lower back,

Geoff Dakin
April 8, 2018
Calgary, AB Canada

Glossary

Adaptive Shortening – a normal physiological process of soft tissue shortening that occurs 24/7 and effects everyone.

Achilles Tendon – also known as the heel cord; a tendon of the back of the leg that attaches the calf to the heel bone.

Ankylosing Spondylitis – chronic inflammatory disease of the spine; bones of spine (and ribcage) fuse together.

Asymmetry – uneven or lacking balance.

Asymptomatic – not pain producing.

Ballistic Stretching – intense stretches that use bouncing movements to force body beyond its normal range of motion

Biomechanical – the application of mechanical principles to living things.

Centrated – optimal, perfectly centered joint position.

Chronic – persisting or lasting for a long time; also, constantly reoccurring.

Compromised – unable to function optimally.

Congenital – a disease or physical abnormality present from birth.

Continuum – a series of almost identical elements that connect two contrasting values (e.g. the line between zero irritation and unbearable irritation).

Contracture – a permanent form of soft tissue shortening

Core Muscles – yes, I know: every therapist talks about 'the core' and strengthening it. So, think of all the muscles between your tailbone and your ribcage. Some experts also consider your glutes to be part of your 'core'.

Debilitating – weakening or to weaken.

Debunk – to show that something is not true.

Dispel – to remove fears, doubts, and/or false ideas.

Dorsiflexion – occurs at the ankle when the toes are brought closer to the shin; think of trying to point toes towards the knee.

Dysfunction – abnormality or impairment in function (usually used to refer to the function of a specified bodily organ or system).

Empirical Evidence – knowledge acquired by means of the senses, particularly by observation and experimentation.

Epidemic – widespread occurrence (usually is used to refer to disease).

Extension – movement by which the bony ends of any joint are drawn away from each other. The angle between the bones increases.

Femur – that's the big bone in your leg, running from your knee to your hip.

Flexion – a bending movement by which the bony ends of any joint are drawn towards each other. The angle between the bones decreases.

Gluteus Medius – one of your three 'glutes'; the medius is situated on the outer surface of your pelvis; it supports your pelvis.

Hamstrings – three muscles on the backside of your thigh; they connect your pelvis to your knee; they oppose your quadriceps.

Hierarchical – an arrangement of items in which the items have a particular order or rank.

Hip Abduction – any movement of the leg away from the midline of your body. Like when you step to the side, get out of bed or get out of the car.

Homeostasis – the tendency of the body to seek and maintain a condition of balance within its internal environment, in spite of external changes.

Hyperextension – the extension of a joint (or joints) beyond normal/healthy limits.

Hyperkyphosis – also known as hunchback, it is an excessive curvature of the upper spine.

Hypermobility – a condition in which the joints move beyond what is considered to be normal/healthy range of motion.

Hypothetical – something that is assumed or based on theory.

Idiopathic – fancy word for 'unknown cause'.

Indelible – something that cannot be removed or forgotten.

Ilium – the two bones on each side of the pelvis (think 'hipbones').

Ischemia – means restricted blood supply.

Lesion – an area of tissue that has been damaged through injury or disease.

Lumbar – the lower part of the back, between the pelvis and the ribs. Right where you are likely to experience lower back pain.

Lymphatic – a circulatory system of vessels (like blood vessels) that carry lymph, an infection fighting fluid, throughout the body.

Misconception – a view or opinion that is incorrect because it is based on faulty thinking or understanding.

Myofascial Trigger Point – a particularly sensitive spot in muscle or connective tissue that when compressed, produces discomfort and "referred sensation" (one or more of a wide variety of sensations, such as heat/cold, numbness/tingling, etc.) in a different location from the trigger point.

Neurological – having to do with the nervous system.

Neuromuscular – having to do with nerves and muscles.

Optimize – to make as effective, perfect, or useful as possible.

Orthotic – pretty much any device that can be used to support bony structures of the body. More often than not, associated with feet or teeth.

Pain-Tension Cycle – a chain of events that creates a state of discomfort. For example, pain causes muscle tension which reduces circulation, which reduces tissue health, which reduces range of motion/creates more discomfort, etc…

Physiologically – having to do with the normal functions of living things.

Plantar Fasciitis – a painful condition most commonly experienced first thing in the morning when getting out of bed. The tissue connecting your heel to your toes in the sole of your foot gets inflamed. Runners often get it. As do people carrying too much weight or wearing improper shoes.

Progression – development toward a destination or a more advanced state, especially involving a gradual evolution through a series of events or stages.

Prone – lying flat, face downward.

Protocol – a set of rules that explain the correct plan and procedures to be followed within a particular system.

Quadriceps – these are the muscles on the front side of your thigh; connecting to your knees, they help you walk, run, jump and squat. They oppose your hamstrings.

Range of Motion – the capacity for movement at a given joint in a specific direction. The anatomy of a joint dictates the normal limits of its range of motion.

Reciprocal Inhibition – a characteristic of our nervous system, where the muscle(s) on one side of a joint relax to accommodate the shortening/contraction of the muscle(s) on the other side. For example, when you straighten your knee by contracting your quadriceps muscles, the muscles responsible for flexion of the knee (your hamstrings) are simultaneously inhibited/relaxed to make that movement of the joint safe and efficient.

Sacrum – that triangular or wedge-shaped bone at the very base of your spine. This pelvic bone sits between your iliums, supports your upper body and connects it to your lower body.

Sciatica – refers to the collection of symptoms (pain, numbness, tingling, weakness) that runs from either the lower back or the glute, down the backside of the leg.

Scoliosis – a sideways curve in the spine.

Supine – lying flat, face upward.

Swayback – a posture that is characterized by the hips pushed too far forward and too much arching in the lower back.

Theoretical Model – a theory designed to explain an entire situation or behavior.

Therapeutic Interventions – actions taken to improve a person's health and well-being.

Vulnerability – to be open or exposed to harm.

Acknowledgements

My first paradigm-shifting experience, as a massage therapist, occurred when I met and studied under Paul St. John. His particular style of neuromuscular therapy blended assessment, manual manipulations and corrective exercise. That may sound typical now, but in the 90's he was a trailblazer. He impressed upon me the importance of pelvic alignment and postural pattern recognition. He's an amazing therapist and I will forever be grateful for his role in my development as a practitioner.

Geoff Gluckman is a corrective-exercise genius. Prior to studying with Geoff, I had used exercise only as a means for strengthening and stabilizing improvements in alignment and function, that had already been obtained via manual manipulations. Geoff demonstrated how you could also use corrective exercise to bring about improvements in alignment and function. That was to be my second paradigm-shifting experience. It gave me a perspective that set me on the path to the evolution of the Alignment First Protocol, which has since allowed me to help tens of thousands of patients, internationally. Thomas Edison famously said, "I start where the last man left off". In my world Geoff Gluckman was that 'last man' and to him I am eternally grateful.

In the mid 90's, Dr. Gordon Hasick proved to me that the position of C1 is the most positionally-important bone in the human body. However, it wasn't until I worked closely with him in 2011, that I discovered the incredible spectrum of ways that malalignment of C1 manifests itself, symptomatically. I learned to make no assumptions about C1 and have now worked with many upper cervical chiropractors over the years, including renowned NUCCA chiropractor Dr. Jeffrey Scholten. I continue to lean on their expertise on a regular basis.

In Chicago, Dr. Evan Osar introduced me to the biomechanical realities, beyond local/global alignment, that have since made me a more complete clinician and prepared me to write this book.

In 2015, I met a referred patient with a complex condition. She was seeing some practitioners I'd already collaborated with, and one I'd never met before. This patient had one of the most difficult pelvic alignment problems I'd ever encountered. At the end of her first session, I told her that, given her circumstances, she was going to wake up tomorrow feeling either amazing or as if she had been hit by a truck. The next morning, she reported she felt "amazing". An hour later, Dr. Curtis Westersund, her neuromuscular dentist, contacted me. Dr. Westersund has become a supporter of my work and a mentor as well. When he's not globetrotting, teaching dentists around the world, he's busy saving the world, one bite at a time.

Dr. Patrick Knott, of the Rosalind Franklin University of Medicine and Science and of Diers Medical Systems, helped me secure Canada's first Diers Body Balance suite of computerized assessment equipment. Not only do we use this hi-tech equipment to make treatment decisions every day; it's helping us understand, on multiple levels, how and why the Alignment First Protocol works.

Finally, Kenneth Gerald Dakin set the bar extremely high in terms of commitment to family, work ethic and integrity. He continues to be my primary benchmark. There's not a day goes by that I don't miss his presence.

Want More?

Head over to www.alignmentfirst.ca and subscribe to my mailing list. It's the best way to keep up-to-date on upcoming books and courses. If you enjoyed this book and found it helpful, please reach out and say "hi" at the clinic, the website or on Facebook. If you leave a candid review on amazon.com, you might just make the difference between someone getting the help they need or not.

"May you live all the days of your life."
— JONATHAN SWIFT

About the Author

Geoff Dakin graduated from the University of British Columbia with an undergraduate degree in Physical Education, in 1987. He then earned a diploma from the West Coast College of Massage Therapy (Vancouver), in 1989.

Early in his career, Geoff recognized that the vast majority of people who suffer with muscle and joint pain also have imbalances in their muscles, postures and movements. The assessment and elimination of these issues have become the heart and soul of his practice, which specializes in treatments based on the principles of his Alignment First Protocol.

A past president of the Massage Therapists Association of British Columbia (MTA of BC), Geoff also spent a year with the Vancouver Canucks in the National Hockey League (1991–92), being one of the first massage therapists in the NHL to travel with his team.

A vocal advocate for the collaborative model of care, Geoff has been working closely with other healthcare specialists to maximize patient success since 1989. He is based in Calgary, Alberta, Canada, where he maintains a private practice. Geoff also coaches massage therapists on how to use his protocol to relieve lower back pain and to help their patients return to an active, healthy lifestyle.

When he's not preserving his patient's independence and mobility and keeping them free from surgery and dependence upon painkillers, Geoff can usually be found with his wife and son, Claudia and Jack. His daughter Vanessa is taking on the world at the University of Victoria, making him proud.

Geoff can be found on Facebook, on his website at alignmentfirst.ca and via email at geoff@alignmentfirst.ca.